MENOPAUSE

MENOPAUSE

A MIDLIFE PASSAGE

EDITED BY

JOAN C. CALLAHAN

INDIANA

UNIVERSITY

PRESS

BLOOMINGTON

AND

INDIANAPOLIS

Hot Flash Fan, fabric construction, by Ann Stewart Anderson in collaboration with fifty-two artists, from the collection of the Kentucky Foundation for Women, Inc. Used by permission of Ann Stewart Anderson and the Kentucky Foundation for Women, Inc. Photograph by Suzanne LaValley.

The paper used in this publication meets the minimum requirements of American National Standard for Information Sciences—Permanence of Paper for Printed Library Materials, ANSI Z39.48-1984.

Manufactured in the United States of America

Library of Congress Cataloging-in-Publication Data

Menopause : a midlife passage / edited by Joan C. Callahan.
        p.   cm.
      Includes bibliographical references and index.
      ISBN 0-253-31312-0 (cloth : alk. paper). — ISBN 0-253-20817-3
(paper : alk. paper)
      1. Menopause—Congresses.   2. Menopause—Social aspects—United
States—Congresses.   3. Menopause—Hormone therapy—Congresses.
I. Callahan, Joan C., date.
RG186.M45   1993
612.6'65—dc20   92-41565

1 2 3 4 5 97 96 95 94 93

For Ronnie

Contents

FOREWORD

CAROLYN S. BRATT

In 1987, three women, members of the Kentucky Commission on Women, were attending a Commission-sponsored conference. All three of the women were in their early forties. All three had been experiencing minor sleep disturbances coupled with vague feelings of uneasiness which did not seem to be related to any external life events. All three of the women were puzzled by these recurring and unfamiliar episodes of insomnia and anxiety. Yet, none of the women had discussed her experiences with anyone else.

During a break in the conference activities, one of the women, with a hint of embarrassment said, "I have been having trouble sleeping at night." The other two women looked at her and nodded slightly. The first woman continued, "I wake up at night with a sense of foreboding, but I don't know why." The other two women looked at each other this time and, again, they both nodded. Hesitantly, one of the other women asked, "Menopause?" The third woman said, "How would we know? If it is menopause, then it's another one of those events in our lives like menstruation, pregnancy, and childbirth that we go through without enough information and that is treated as an illness." The other women nodded their agreement. That conversation was the catalyst for a series of events that have culminated in this book.

The tentative conversation of these three women soon expanded into more formalized discussions with other women about menopause. Some members of this ad hoc group of "femmes d'une certaine age" were on faculty at the University of Kentucky in anthropology, art history, law, nursing, philosophy, sociology, and theater. One group member was an elected officeholder. Other members were involved in issues affecting Appalachian or African-American women. An endocrinologist and an internist also joined the group.

A consensus eventually emerged from the group's discussions. The group realized that most women possess little accurate information about menopause because stereotyped menopausal images and biased information about menopausal changes are a widespread and persistent part of our culture. Also, many women have few or no discussions with their mothers or older female relatives because of a shared reluctance to discuss this common experience in the lives of women. The arts and literature do not provide assistance in understanding the menopausal experience because they contain only a few, usually negative, images of and reflections upon menopause. Finally, much of the contemporary research on menopause takes place within either a biomedical framework that approaches menopause as a disease or a social paradigm that interprets menopause solely as a social, cultural, or symbolic event. The group came to understand that neither approach adequately captures the complex and multifaceted nature of women's menopausal experience.

In order to share with other women their growing understanding of menopause as a universal developmental event, the group decided to sponsor a conference on menopause for women in the Southeast region, academicians, and professionals. One conference goal was to help remedy the paucity of information available to women about menopause by providing a forum for the dissemination of current information. A second goal of the conference planning group was to help counter the trend toward making menopause another medicalized event in women's lives. To accomplish its third goal of increasing the actual body of information on menopause, the planning group envisioned a conference that would encourage new approaches to scholarly research on the menopausal experience.

The planning group sought to achieve its goals by ensuring diversity both in the conference presentations and in the audience. Presentations on menopause were systematically solicited from the social sciences, humanities, visual and performing arts, and the health professions. In addition to encouraging conference attendance by those who had a professional interest in the topic, the planning group tried to ensure that women who had a personal interest in menopause would attend, too. To that end, the planning group imposed a common requirement on all conference presenters. In a radical departure from the traditional, specialized academic conference, all of the conference presentations had to be accessible to nonspecialists.

What finally materialized was a multidisciplinary, multidimensional conference on menopause which drew a standing-room-only crowd of more than 300 participants. Cross-cultural, biological, artistic, and transhistorical perspectives on menopause were included in the conference program. For example, Ann Stewart Anderson, an artist, presented visual images of menopause from her "Hot Flash" series of paintings and displayed as well as discussed the creation of her fabric piece, *Hot Flash Fan*. Joy Webster Barbre traced the historical evolution of American perspectives of menopause. As part of a panel of experts, Mary Lou Logothetis, Kristi J. Ferguson, and Kathleen I. MacPherson explored the diversity and complexity of opinions on the value of HRT (hormone replacement therapy) for menopausal women.

Perhaps the most important segments of the conference were the two which permitted the unmediated voices of individual women to be heard. Letters describing personal menopausal experiences and intergenerational messages were solicited from postmenopausal women. These letters and messages were displayed at the conference. Informal opportunities were provided for conference participants to share their responses to the correspondence. A video production was developed and shown as a work-in-progress at the conference. Kentucky women from different geographical, cultural, racial, ethnic, educational, and economic backgrounds were filmed as they talked about their own and their mothers' experiences with menopause.

As another part of the planning group's attempt to ensure the participation of regional women in the conference, a decision was made to invite a nationally known keynote speaker. However, identifying such a person seemed problematic after more than a year of discussions within the group failed to identify a nationally known "expert" on menopause. Finally, the committee realized that the paucity of information on menopause explained the fact that there was no well-known "expert" to recruit as the keynote speaker.

The planning group then realized that the question was not who is a nationally recognizable expert on menopause. The correctly formulated question was: Who would women want to hear reflecting on the menopausal experience? One name came quickly to mind—Susan Stamberg of National Public Radio. Ms. Stamberg was contacted, and she immediately accepted the invitation. She did not disappoint the planning group or her audience. Her keynote address on being a menopausal woman provided the same insightful, and often humorous, commentary that we all had come to expect from her work as cohost of "All Things Considered" and later as host of "Weekend Edition."

The ad hoc planning group that put together the "Menopause: A Midlife Passage" conference no longer meets on a regular basis, but each member continues to pursue her individual and professional interest in the menopausal experience. Our hope is that this book of essays will be a part of a continuing, innovative dialogue about menopause rather than merely the conclusion of the conversation begun by those three women more than five years ago.

ACKNOWLEDGMENTS

No book is ever the result of a single person's efforts. That is so much more true when there are a number of authors who create a new work. The contributors to this volume have been an editor's dream, and I can never thank them adequately for their commitment to the project and for their trust and patience through several unforeseeable delays. Special thanks are due to contributors Geri L. Dickson, Jean Kozlowski, Patricia Smith, and Ann M. Voda, who were not part of the conference with which the collection began, but who accepted my invitation to contribute original essays to the volume, despite enormous demands on their time from other quarters. I am doubly grateful to Ann Stewart Anderson for permission to use her work.

And, once again, I have substantially increased my debts to Jennifer Crossen for everything from sustained enthusiasm for the project, through helpful substantive suggestions, to proofreading—all cheerfully made time for, despite the demands of a six-year-old, myriad dogs and cats, thirty horses, countless riding students, and a consistent running program. I hesitate to remind her . . .

As the Foreword and Introduction indicate, this collection grew out of the interest of a group of women in learning more about menopause. Each of these women played a significant role in making the conference that began this book a reality. Thanks, then, to Susan Abbott, Carolyn S. Bratt, Paula Fletcher, Bev Futrell, Betty Gabehart, Karen Greenwell, Chris Havice, Jo Hendrix, Gretchen LaGodna, Sally Maggard, Paula Maionchi, Gerri Maschio, Debra Merchant, Pam Miller, and Josephine Richardson, who were on the conference planning committee, and to Lynda Charles, who so efficiently managed the many logistical details of the conference. And for joining in so many of the planning meetings, special thanks to Karen Jones of Lexington's own and incomparable Reel World String Band (Flying Fish Records), from which we also borrowed Bev Futrell for the planning committee.

Double thanks are due to Paula Fletcher, who not only worked with us on the planning committee, but who also did the conference presentation on the physiology of menopause; and to Chris Havice, who prepared an illuminating slide presentation on the representation of midlife women in art and who brought us Ann Stewart Anderson's wonderful *Hot Flash Fan*. And triple thanks are due to Carolyn S. Bratt, who enlisted Susan Stamberg as our keynote speaker; to Gretchen LaGodna, for her remarkable series of taped conversations with women discussing menopause, which added so much to the conference; and to Carolyn and Gretchen together, who found the funding and made it all happen.

The conference would not have been possible without the generous support of Sallie Bingham, the Kentucky Commission on Women, the Kentucky Humanities Council, the University of Kentucky Office of Research and Graduate Studies, the University of Kentucky Medical Center Office for Research and Graduate Studies, and the University of Kentucky College of Medicine. Additional thanks to the Kentucky Foundation for Women, Inc., for lending us the *Hot Flash Fan* for the conference and for permission to use its image in the book's afterword.

Warm thanks to our inspired and patient photographer, Aimee Tomasek, and to everyone (including the pets) who participated in our "power surge" photo session for the book's cover: Carlotta Abbott, Susan Abbott (and Sausage), Anita Bolen, Anna Bosch, Carolyn Bratt, Joan Catapano, Betsy Churchill, Debra Claus-Walker, Lenore R. Cole, Anne-Bennett Cook, Marilyn Cook, Willa Crabtree, David Crossen, Jennifer Crossen, Susan Faupel, Susan Michele Frain, Bev Futrell, Betty Gabehart, Gloria Gellin, Lillian Gentry, Mary Beth Haas, Laura C. Harris, Chris Havice, LuAnne Clark Holladay, Beth C. Israel, Karen Jones, Laura Kaplan, Linda LaPorte (and Credit), Geri Maschio, Mary McKenna (and Lady), Susan Scollay, Barb Sherrer, Ronnie Sheehy, Sue Strong, Rose Thiedich, and Karen Tice. Our banner is the product of heroic graphic design work by Susie Hull and staff. Finally, very special thanks must go to my generous colleague, Jim Force, who so enthusiastically provided his prized 1969 Buick Electra 225 convertible, and to the women of Ferne Sales and Manufacturing of West Orange, New Jersey, for permission to use their bumper sticker and its message that "they are not hot flashes . . . they are power surges."

The book is dedicated to Ronnie Sheehy, in unsayable thanks for her lifelong friendship and infinitely good-natured grace through everything, including menopause.

Proceeds from this volume will go to the Women's Studies Program at the University of Kentucky.

INTRODUCTION

JOAN C. CALLAHAN

In 1988, at the suggestion of Carolyn S. Bratt, a group of sixteen women from Kentucky and Ohio began meeting to discuss menopause. We quickly began to consider the possible value of organizing a multidisciplinary conference on menopause. Most of us knew very little about menopause, and we thought that bringing together people from a variety of backgrounds and perspectives would provide us with a much-needed education. At the same time, we realized that if we were so underinformed about menopause, it was probable that many women were equally underinformed and that a conference on the topic that was open to the public would likely be helpful to a number of women in our geographical area.

After meeting for several months to discuss the shape such a conference might take, we decided that we wanted a program that would raise and offer reflection on some of the central personal, cultural, medical, conceptual, moral, and public policy issues that are raised for women by menopause and, more generally, by midlife. To this end, we invited some papers and put out a call for papers that reached health care providers, medical and social scientists, philosophers, artists, and feminists from all disciplines. The conference (which quickly filled to our capacity of 325) took place in the fall of 1989, and the core of this collection is comprised of updated essays selected from the conference papers. This core has been supplemented with several additional papers invited for the collection.

Like the conference, the purpose of this collection is to add to the public understanding of menopause and the position of midlife women. Within this general purpose, the primary goal of the book is to articulate and offer some substantive reflection on differing perspectives on menopause and women's midlife as they appear in various cultural quarters and among women. In service of this goal, the papers come from social scientists, who elucidate some cultural and personal perspectives on menopause; health care researchers and providers who explain the physiology of menopause, who explain how menopause has become a medicalized phenomenon in the United States, who examine the biases underpinning menopause research, and who discuss the current disagreements regarding the safety and efficacy of hormone replacement therapy (HRT); an artist, whose work has recently focused on women's highly textured experience of menopause; a screeplay author and film critic, who discusses the representation of midlife women in film and opportunities in film for midlife women; and philosophers and policy analysts who help to clarify some of the central conceptual, moral, and policy questions raised by menopause. Part I of the collection focuses on cultural constructions of women's midlife and menopause, the assumptions underlying those constructions, and some of the implications of those constructions in current social practices. Part II focuses on providing a careful discussion of the HRT debate and a clear description of the physiology and endocrinology of menopause.

More particularly: Since the influence of film is so pervasive in contemporary society, the collection opens with Jean Kozlowski's "Women, Film, and the Midlife Sophie's Choice: Sink or Sousatzka?" which explores the treatment of midlife women in contemporary film, along with the troublesomely limited and stereotypical choices the film industry commonly offers actresses at midlife. Kozlowski points out that at midlife actresses are forced into a "'Sophie's Choice' . . . between fading into early retirement or accepting unglamorous, eccentric, prematurely elderly roles . . . which . . . are . . . insulting to real-life elderly women. . . . " This neutralization of the midlife woman, says Kozlowski, "is both a sexist insult and a dirty trick," which forces no longer fertile but still fully vibrant women into self-betrayal by precluding opportunities for them to represent that vibrancy on film. Kozlowski finishes with the warning that we "can't afford to acquiesce in the continued devaluation of ourselves in a medium that interprets our lives and has the potential to shape generations."

The location of woman's value and vibrancy in her reproductive capacities is taken up by Joy Webster Barbre in "Meno-Boomers and Moral Guardians: An Exploration of the Cultural Construction of Menopause." Barbre points out that despite marked differences in the Victorian and contemporary American perspectives on women, there are significant similarities between those perspectives, which are rooted in a common view of the importance of women's reproductive capacities to understanding the nature and value of women. Barbre's paper ends by raising the question of whether recent scientific work on menopause and the "rush to save [women] from menopause" rests on questionable assumptions regarding women's biology, women's appropriate social roles, women's aging, and prevailing social values.

Barbre's paper raises the issue of perceptions of menopause as disease and the question of the appropriateness of the medicalization of menopause. Geri L. Dickson's "Metaphors of Menopause: The Metalanguage of Menopause Research" explores this question further by describing four paradigms that have underpinned menopause research (biomedical, sociocultural, feminist, and postmodern paradigms) and each of their assumptions about science, women, and the "reality" of menopause. Reminiscent of Barbre and particularly anticipatory of the papers by Mary Lou Logothetis and Rosalind Ekman Ladd, Dickson challenges the biomedical conceptualization of menopause, while calling for a recognition that our science has been perspective-laden in a way that fails to take into account the full range of experiences, attitudes, and responses of women in regard to menopause.

Continuing the discussion of conceptual deconstruction begun by Dickson and anticipating Jill Rips's discussion of categorizations, Jacquelyn N. Zita's "Heresy in the Female Body: The Rhetorics of Menopause" shows how menopause has been seen as a "heresy" in the female body. She describes three ways in which menopause is currently rhetoricized, showing how each of these rhetorics presupposes a different view of female embodiment, and the consequences for women of these different views. Zita ends by calling for continued work on removing demeaning gender biases from the interpretation of menopause, on improving the material circumstances of postmenopausal women, and on eliminating in the culture a metaphysical misogyny that is intolerant of the crone, thereby making way for women to be "more powerful . . . unruly . . . old, wise, and furiously heretical."

Continuing the discussion of conceptual classifications begun by Barbre and carried through by Dickson and Zita, Jill Rips's "Who Needs a Menopause Policy?" explores some questions of menopause and public policy. Rips focuses on the question of whether a feminist perspective on menopause should issue in recommendations for policies that specifically address the needs of menopausal women. Following Zita's explicit call for attention to the well-being of women, she asks whether public policies set up to serve needs of menopausal women are likely to serve women well. This question leads Rips to explore some problems created by categorizations in general and by the categorization of women as menopausal in particular, and she concludes that public policies established for the sake of menopausal women as such may, in fact, militate against the interests of women.

Patricia Smith's "Selfish Genes and Maternal Myths: A Look at Postmenopausal Pregnancy" continues Rips's discussion of practice and what is *really* in the interests of women. Smith explores a number of intriguing questions that combine over what might be described as the ultimate rejection of the postmenopausal woman—medical technology's brand new capacity to make postmenopausal women pregnant. Smith's central questions pertain to why a postmenopausal woman might want to deploy this technology. In exploring the most plausible answers, she argues that postmenopausal pregnancy serves the interests of neither women nor children well, and that this technology, like others before it, continues to tie the value of women to reproductive capacity—precisely the value rejected by Kozlowski's opening paper.

The biomedical construction of menopause discussed through the papers in Part I is intimately linked to the current debate over hormone replacement therapy (HRT), which is the focus of Part II.

HRT has become widely prescribed in recent years; yet many women are disinclined to accept it. Continuing discussion of the medicalization of menopause and the question of women's experience of and responses to menopause begun in Part I, Mary Lou Logothetis's "Disease or Development: Women's Perceptions of Menopause and the Need for Hormone Replacement Therapy" explores women's attitudes toward menopause and toward their need for HRT. Her study reveals that many women (indeed ninety percent of the women in her sample) have quite positive attitudes toward menopause. At the same time, and for various reasons, not the least of which is disagreement over HRT in the medical community, many women are highly ambivalent about accepting HRT.

The reasons for disagreement over the safety and efficacy of HRT are articulated and explored in "Making a Reasoned Choice about Hormone Replacement Therapy," by Susan R. Johnson and Kristi J. Ferguson, and in "The False Promises of Hormone Replacement Therapy and Current Dilemmas," by Kathleen I. MacPherson. These papers, respectively, clearly elucidate the central arguments for and the central arguments against use of HRT.

In "A Journey to the Center of the Cell: Understanding the Physiology and Endocrinology of Menopause," Ann M. Voda continues the discussion of the mythology of menopause found throughout the papers in Part I, and she explains the physical changes that comprise menopause and that these changes are the normal effects of withdrawal from estrogen rather than symptoms of disease. Voda also explains the specific effects of exogenous hormones on the cell, why hormone use has been associated with various untoward side effects, and what open questions remain about hormone therapies. Like MacPherson, Voda concludes that the case against widespread use of HRT overwhelms the case supporting it.

Given the current state of disagreement over HRT, women's informed consent to HRT is a matter of the most serious moral concern. Rosalind Ekman Ladd's "Medical Decision Making: Issues Concerning Menopause" concludes Part II with a discussion of this issue and, more generally, with a discussion of the treatment of menopause-age women by health care practitioners. Ladd emphasizes the uncertainty of clinical judgment in this area, and she argues for the primacy of women's involvement in decisions regarding accepting HRT, echoing Johnson and Ferguson's insistence that women need to make themselves as knowledgeable as possible before making a decision about hormone replacement.

Bringing us back to the arts in the Afterword, Ann Stewart Anderson's "Creating a Visual Image of Menopause: The *Hot Flash Fan*," describes the creation of the genuinely unique and cooperatively created fabric piece, the *Hot Flash Fan*, which depicts the great variety of experiences, perceptions, and states women associate with menopause. An image of the *Fan* appears in the afterword to this volume.

Finally, Jill Rips brings the collection to a conclusion with a selected interdisciplinary bibliography on menopause.

This book has been a women's cooperative project from its conceptualization through its completion. We all hope that it will help in making common, at last, a deeper, more textured, and hence, more appropriate understanding of women's menopause as a midlife passage.

Windy Knoll Farm
Lexington, Kentucky
June 1992

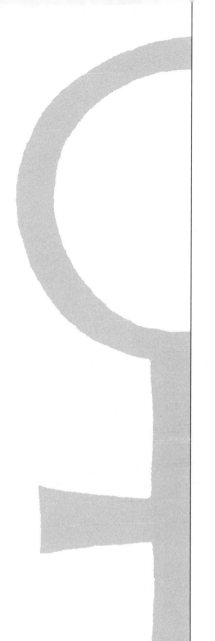

Part
One

Cultural
Constructions,
Policy, and
Practice

Women, Film, and the Midlife Sophie's Choice: Sink or Sousatzka?

Jean Kozlowski

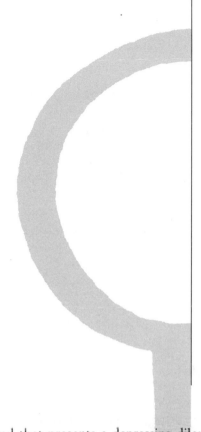

Something is happening to Shirley MacLaine, which rhymes with *What Ever Happened to Baby Jane?* and spells the same kind of trouble. Although not entirely her fault, she's surrendering too willingly, and that presents a depressing dilemma to other women facing the midpoint of our lives. Since our society seems to demand a distinct, preferably exaggerated transition for women from "youth" to "maturity" (read "obsolescence"), what's happening to MacLaine represents more than a forced tradeoff that middle-aged actresses accept in order to stay visible and keep their hats in the Hollywood ring. It's a surrender that cheats all of us looking for positive role models for maintaining viable postyouth identities in a callously youth-driven culture.

MacLaine waved the white flag in 1988 with *Madame Sousatzka,* a film which by her own admission launched her career into the realm of character acting, far from the frenzied transience of the "youth market." She went out of her way in interviews coinciding with the film's release to give the impression that it was she who was calling the shots in this choice; that the social norm which renders women her age uninteresting and, consequently, invisible was a nonissue. "I had to pry myself away from the priorities of cosmetic vanity," she told film critic Roger Ebert (1–2). "It was time to stop taking parts that are traditional leading lady movie-star showcases, and rather take the parts that are questionable and dangerous but wonderful, parts that you can get into." Sounding like protesting too much, talking herself as much as any viewer into accepting this discomfiting new persona, such statements come across like defense mechanisms against the humiliation of being stripped of power and purpose, as if no longer being young is a debilitating deficiency disease.

Ebert apparently didn't ask the obvious questions about why there must be a "time" for women to stop being the central focus of a story or why leading lady vehicles and more "dangerous," "wonderful" roles must be mutually exclusive. One can speculate on whether or not he overlooked the important underlying issues here because, as a man, he's a member of the dominant group in our culture and as such will never suffer from a lack of fair or adequate images to relate to at any stage of his life. In this case, what's left unsaid virtually shouts the truth about how women at midlife are perceived.

MacLaine gave a gutsy performance as the antiquated Sousatzka, but then "gutsy" is a safe word to use when something is as disconcerting as it is touching. Granted, it takes a certain amount of artistic bravery to earn the (debatable) accolade, but for women this often means a bold leap past character acting, straight into caricature. And for women of a certain age, such a move translates into a kind of celluloid death wish, an often irrevocable toying with fascinated revulsion in an audience taken aback. MacLaine herself acknowledged that the appeal of *Madame Sousatzka* might be limited to those who "want to go see how Shirley has turned into a ruin. . . . You might want to go like you go watch an accident."

This is an interesting and, given the cultural obsoletism that oppresses women as we age, revealing attitude. Maybe we need a word like "gutsy" to help put the best light on witnessing a startling sellout. Shirley MacLaine has made a point of coming across otherwise as a lively, accomplished woman who, still strutting her stuff on a Vegas stage, could have shown us with gleeful pride what fiftysomething looks like. Madame Sousatzka isn't it.

For women over fifty, the transition to character acting may be construed as not so much a tour de force challenge as a bite-the-bullet rite of passage that, like our youth-culture's view of menopause, signals the end of productivity. With limited opportunities to practice the craft they've spent much of their lives honing, their "Sophie's choice" is between fading into early retirement or accepting unglamorous, eccentric, prematurely elderly roles (which, generally unflattering, are in turn insulting to real-life elderly women); ceding leading lady appeal to younger women whose mothers, aunts, and grandmothers they will play. This is both a sexist insult and a dirty trick.

Men don't get neutralized this way. Robert Redford, Burt Reynolds, and Clint Eastwood (not to mention Warren Beatty) are not expected to submit to a ritualized "graduation" past leading man status into keeping their careers afloat by playing oddball curmudgeons. Jack Nicholson's ebbing hairline and swelling waistline won't downgrade his box office appeal. Chances are good that, within the next several years, Robert De Niro won't be placing a bitingly pointed ad in *Variety* to remind the industry he's still kicking, as fifty-four-year-old Bette Davis did in 1962: "Thirty years experience as an actress in motion pictures. Mobile still and more affable than rumor would have it. Wants steady employment in Hollywood" (Stine with Davis 310–11). When De Niro (born in 1943) told "Entertainment Tonight" that he wanted, at that point in his life, to "work a lot," there was no doubt that opportunities would be plentiful and no reservation that, now that he'd played a mental patient (*Awakenings,* 1990), he'd made a fateful "transition" that would preclude his return to slicker leading roles. He and the others are part of a more flexible market, on the right side of the double standard that also easily sells older character actors as romantic leads. Gene Hackman said at age sixty-one that he was thinking of slowing down; three films a year is a bit hectic. It would be interesting to know how many leads, romantic or otherwise, Shirley MacLaine has been asked to consider since entering this phase of her career with *Madame Sousatzka*.

The dirty trick for women is that marketability is not guaranteed by the transition to character roles. As statistics presented at the 1990 Screen Actors Guild Women's Conference made obvious, with nearly 71 percent of all SAG feature film roles going to men, there's a paucity of good women's roles, particularly for actresses in their forties, fifties, and sixties—the peak earning years for men (Dawes 3). But there's also a limit to the number of Sousatzkas the public will flock to see; a short statute of limitations before a bravura risk degenerates into cliché and the maverick soul becomes the generic "loony old bag," a minor role hardly designed to carry a film. Eventually even performers of Ellen Burstyn's caliber are reduced to nothing-part Nurse Ratched rehashes in TV fare like *When You Remember Me* (1990); wasted in throwaways like the somehow inevitable TV remake of *What Ever Happened to Baby Jane?* (1991), starring Vanessa and Lynn Redgrave. We've likewise seen Anne Bancroft's and Joanne Woodward's considerable talent underused in recent years, Bancroft having gone directly from vamping Tim Matheson in *To Be or Not To Be* 1983) to a stint in typecasting—a parade of nagging mamas in *Garbo Talks* (1984), *'night Mother* (1986), and *Torch Song Trilogy* (1988), with only roles as a Mother Superior nun in *Agnes of God* (1985) and as an author/

correspondent in *84, Charing Cross Road* (1987) varying the march. It remains to be seen whether Woodward will reemerge with new marketability thanks to her Best Actress Oscar nomination for *Mr. and Mrs. Bridge* (1990).

But how much latitude will having triumphed in what is for the most part a "safely sixtyish" role allow her? Could she, for example, now choose to do a love story opposite, say, Mel Gibson? After all, there's almost the same age gap between Sean Connery and Michelle Pfeiffer in *The Russia House* (1990), yet this pairing hardly raised eyebrows. The difference here, however, swings in the traditionally "proper" direction—toward the man, who can play lover or father, feel young again as he controls the situation either way, and reaffirm his potency with a still-fertile female who, unlike a more mature woman, will be impressed by and defer to his experience and wisdom. In men, as Elissa Melamed points out, the aging process is associated with a buildup of power, while aging women are dismissed as "over the hill" (78). At issue is the ability to produce, which in American male terms has always meant a capacity to wield socioeconomic power and carries a connotation of youthfulness (Melamed 40, 60–61). The flipside for American women is a simplistic, anatomy-is-destiny-based correlation between reproductive capability and personal worth.

It's this notion of female fertility that's the primary deciding factor in how women are depicted in film and how we end up regarding ourselves within our life cycles and our social environment. It's a cunningly effective standard simply because it has become so deeply ingrained that, from the filmmakers who reinforce it to the women who accept it, its validity has gone largely unquestioned. We all know that middle-aged women today lead productive lives, are more health- and fitness-conscious, and do not dress like truant officers in *Our Gang* comedies. But in film they're still summarily dismissed as dotty, overbearing busybodies and frustrated, repressed victims of their own change-of-life dementia. We've been taught to laugh at them as targets of mother-hatred and as exemplars of all that is no longer sexually desirable. We're out of luck if we're looking for realistic, affirmative touchstones. Movies tend to give us only an abrupt shove from cute ingenue to weird old crone (without the respected wise woman connotation the word originally had). All we come away with is a cartoon image of the acceptable screen woman—an amazing special-effects creature who beneath her nubile jiggle or her craggy makeup is missing the entire midsection of her life. Sooner or later it has to dawn on us that something is definitely wrong with this picture.

The fertility criterion is not a female construct; it reflects incredibly skewed reasoning that can't possibly be based on women's reality. We are not the ones who, from the earliest days of human history, when observations of nature led to a veneration of women's seemingly magical kinship with the earth in the ability to create new life, felt threatened by female "power." We didn't go out of our way to construct a rigidly linear, patriarchal religious system that dictated a denial and debasement of the very forces and cycles our bodies seemed to represent. We have, nonetheless, spent centuries seeing ourselves through male eyes, with near-sighted masculine vision that perceives objects only in direct relation to the observing male's ego and obliterates whatever is mystifying, enviable, frightening, and/or can't be appropriated for the viewer's use. No man can "achieve" childbearing, although the image switch from the primeval earth mother whose "wise blood" alone made babies (Walker [1985] 1988, 20) to the medieval woman-as-vessel who merely incubated the man's "homunculus" (Sjöö and Mor 278) was a nice try. Menstruation can't be coopted, though anthropological evidence suggests men have tried to do so through their own genital-bloodletting rituals (Sjöö and Mor 184; Walker [1985] 1988, 47–49). Women's film images, on the other hand, can be and, by virtue of male control of the industry, have been wrenched away from the truth of our own experience as women to become what Jean Baker Miller terms the dominant group's inevitable description of a subordinate group in false terms derived from its own systems of thought (xix). Since film is an insidiously powerful tool for telling us what we aren't as women and what we should be—always with men's best interests in mind, of course—what we *are* is controlled by an annihilation of self-esteem that comes to us, like a spoonful of sugar helping the medicine go down, in the form of entertainment. So, conditioned for shame about our bodies as they age, we watch portraits of once-vital women degenerate before our eyes while the men they support, each his own Dorian Gray, retain supernatural youthfulness. And yet we are somehow the evil ones, evoking a terror that on close examination is really a projection of men's fear of mortality and dependency on women.

That women's film images are arrested at precisely the point at which men are attaining peak socioeconomic status is more than a modern assertion of male superiority. Middle age is for both sexes a time of taking stock, which, in a positive light, comprises concepts of further growth and development amenable to conscious life reshaping (Butler 1943) when opportunity and resources allow. But not all women have access to alternatives at midlife, and our self-inventory of life role satisfaction (Barnett 53) isn't considered important, anyway. Often, then, since men's interests dominate the media, the images we see (and don't see) provide clues to their anxiety that, under it all, the success and the power, life is slipping by. An aging woman may be a keen reminder of this and find herself a lightning rod for male resentment.

Then there's always the threat that we might at menopause discover freedom long suppressed through years of childrearing and housewifery and use it to our advantage. Should that happen, the entire patriarchal superstructure, which since the god concept got a sex change and went macho has depended on women's subservience, would collapse. Men are quick to turn our biological "facts" against us, and yet the significant implications of postmenopausal potential have been ignored—or suppressed. As psychiatrist Anne M. Seiden has noted (1000), menopause is a distinctly human characteristic favored by natural selection to allow a woman a number of years of freedom from new pregnancies to pursue other activities. Whether in regard to pursuing personal interests or to becoming breadwinners, through necessity or desire, this belies the "it's all over" epitaph we're supposed to carry into midlife and opens horizons we haven't been encouraged to consider. How many men want to open that Pandora's box on film, put ideas into our heads? Better to ignore us 'til we're "safely elderly" and less likely to embark on journeys of self-discovery, and more apt to dote on than challenge them intellectually, emotionally, socially, or sexually. Granny roles in Hollywood are then a welcome mat for the returning prodigal daughter exiled for her midlife hormonal upheaval.

Which begs a question about exactly where men see themselves while we're going through all these supposedly degenerative changes. Melamed postulates that the male conceives of his body as "stable" as opposed to the changeability of the female body through childbearing, menstruation, and menopause (35–36). Change for men is frequently negative; not cyclical, but linear, leading to a waning of power and eventual death, and without a comfortable sense of aging as part of the life cycle. The trick, then, is to deny change, perhaps by surrounding oneself with a semblance of youth—in the form of younger partners. This idea of bodily continuity, in addition to establishing a male-oriented standard that casts female differences as liabilities, (Melamed 36) can be stretched into a fantasy of ageless sexual potency. Hence, through the hoodoo of, not just film, but social conditioning, Sean Connery is welcome to Michelle Pfeiffer on screen, and at age sixty to the cover of the 18 December 1989 issue of *People* Magazine as "The Sexiest Man Alive."

The same phenomenon maintained Clark Gable as a sex symbol way past the shelf life any woman's physical appeal would be granted. Nowhere is this better exemplified than in the film he made twice: *Red Dust* (1932), reborn in 1953 as *Mogambo*. In *Red Dust*, thirty-one-year-old Gable, all sassy manliness and dangerous charm, grouses that women— especially white women who "can't stand the gaffe"—don't belong in his he-man, Indochinese domain. Whereupon he and twenty-one-year-old interloper Jean Harlow—a very white woman with a shady past—have a gritty, buddy-buddy fling that, while often patronizing (his calling her "kid" exceeds '30s colloquialism to make it clear he has the upper hand in this situational diversion), mixes a chemistry of counterparts for a believable sizzle or two. Enter Mary Astor, at twenty-six the virtuous married woman whom Gable genuinely falls for, and the triangle constructs itself along lines made volatile by credible sexual and moral tension.

Play the same story out again in Africa, twenty-one years later, and the fantasy that the male side of the triangle is the constant in the design—the immutable base which, combined with interchangeable female supports, still forms a compelling configuration—fizzles. *Mogambo*'s Gable is fifty-two and hasn't entirely kept a grip on that "bodily stability" of male mythology. He spends most of the movie looking dazedly introspective, as if he himself has had trouble "standing the gaffe." What had a scrappy chumminess in 1932 looks avuncular at best in 1953; when he calls thirty-year-old Ava Gardner, cast in the Harlow role, "kid," it's as if he means her to go play in the jungle and leave him alone. (For a startling sense of how much time elapsed between these films, Gardner in her autobiography recalls swooning, at age nine, over Gable in the very film she'd grow up to make over with him [178].)

Perhaps some of the hesitancy in this film can be blamed on 1950s anal retentive morality; perhaps some of it is simply a lack of sparks between the actors. Gardner radiates a plucky warmth as a woman with a single event in her life—the wartime death of her husband—to explain the "scars" she now bears and her descent into fallen womanhood. The bloom is not so far off the rose as to render her a dried old blossom; the reputation not so tarnished that Gable's interest in her, at least theoretically, can't buff the youthful sheen back up. It doesn't matter if he appears not quite up to the task; the fact that she wants him is supposed to obviate the necessity of his having to prove himself. Grace Kelly at twenty-five had the Astor role, but her peculiar acting style—a sort of histrionic woodenness—only increased the distance between the characters. Certainly she was lovely—in sexist ideology and Hollywood shorthand an appropriate prize for an ailing, aging male ego. The ads for the movie that blazoned, "They fought like sleek jungle cats! . . . The jungle strips two civilized women of all but their most primeval instincts!" (Gardner 179) left no doubt that it was intended to appeal not to women fantasizing about Gable, but to men identifying with him as the Great White Hunter bagging hot feline quarry. One critic's cartwheeling praise, with words like "socko," "sizzling," and "sexy two-fisted adventure" (*Variety Film Reviews*), proves how well the conceit worked.

When a man reaches his middle years and needs the reassurance that he's still "got it," pairing him with a woman who's his equal in terms of life experience is tantamount to holding up a mirror to reveal his own mortality. Additionally, if he sees his female peer as the same age his mother was when he was endeavoring to break away from her and begin his manhood adventures, his overriding impulse may be to run like hell. If he happens to be a film-maker, he can flee by cooking up images to keep women his age in their place as he most negatively remembers it: they're mothers, not playmates. And, like little boys who imagine their big, bad mommies as evil witches, he can conjure up an archetypal association of women's power over him with nature's destructive forces and turn them into withered harridans he has a right to escape. It then becomes incumbent upon actresses reaching this age he sees as dangerous to accept and disseminate these stereotypes. If they want to keep working.

Economic considerations are seldom cited in the decisions middle-aged actresses make to accept parts that don't necessarily make the best use of their talents. In this respect, Hollywood is no different from society at large for women seeking security against the threat of being cast aside. Mary Astor was forty-seven in 1953, but it would have been conventionally inappropriate to the illusion and defeated the purpose of the remake to reunite her with Gable in *Mogambo*. She'd by then signed a long-term contract with Metro-Goldwyn-Mayer for security's sake and promptly found herself being railroaded down the studio's idea of the "mommy track." In 1938 she was cast as teenager Judy Garland's mother in *Listen Darling*, the first of what she called a "long career of Mothers for Metro" (Astor 141). Being nudged toward eventual "Sousatzkadom" did not sit well with her: "I was in my late thirties and it played hell with my image of myself" (171). By the time she starred as Marmee in *Little Women* (1949), she was concurrently experiencing difficult early symptoms of a problematic menopause and starved for recognition as something more than the quintessential personification of movie motherhood. "I was not an unattractive woman," she declared by male-standard way of assessing her potential (194). "O.K., I'd play all the mothers they wanted: the selfish, domineering mother; the warm, understanding mother. Mother. M.O.T.H.E.R. Fine. But there wasn't a mother in every script, and was I to sit around until there was?" While shooting *Little Women,* she sought relief from the claustrophobia of her image by moonlighting across the lot on another set (in *Act of Violence*), playing Marmee's polar opposite: "a sleazy, aging whore" (199). "It was such a contrast," she said, "that it was stimulating and reviving."

Yet what kind of victory is it for a woman to go from being seen as the mature madonna keeping the home fires burning while her man is at war to an overused commodity long past lighting men's sexual fires? It would be tough to find a more succinctly revelatory film symbol of men's ambivalence toward the menopausal woman than one actress delineating both extremes simultaneously.

Such stereotypes negate our complexity as human beings whether we're young women identified by body parts and hair color ("a leggy blonde," "a busty redhead") or older women categorized by time's effect on our relation to men ("an aging sex goddess," "a lonely spinster"). The extremes provide an orderly code by which men can peg us quickly and avoid venturing into the increasingly unfamiliar depths of our characters as our journey through womanhood changes us. As with any sea, the most perilous currents occur not on the shores of embarkation or destination, but at midpoint, where a man can find himself cast adrift and helpless. How telling that this is precisely the part of our adventure that Hollywood imagemakers most insistently choose to downplay.

From what we see, then—and again, more importantly, *don't* see— we're led to conclude that midlife women are inappreciable bores. We get spoon-fed multidimensional character studies of every kind of fiftyish male, from backwoods good ol' boys to regular joes toughing it out in the big city, ad nauseam. Their female counterparts are extremely rare and must be either twice as extraordinary or endure brutal victimization to earn equivalent attention. This is a familiar picture of women's reality in our society. And Hollywood betrays its image as a cultural mover and shaker when it refuses to promote strong, positive, sensitive portraits of mature women.

Changing this won't be possible as long as middle age functions as the perfect setting for a male morality play about women's treacherous nature. Vivien Leigh, whom men knew precisely how to relate to as Scarlett O'Hara or Blanche DuBois, entered murkier waters when she turned forty-seven and took on another Tennessee Williams character, Karen

Stone, in *The Roman Spring of Mrs. Stone* (1960). A recently widowed stage actress forced to realize she's past playing Shakespearean ingenues, Mrs. Stone decides she has no talent (i.e., she's obsolete), and promptly retires. (While the message here to older women is obvious, the assumption that there are no other roles she could take is unfortunately more credible than the script likely intended). Once self-exiled to Rome, she gets entangled with pouty gigolo Warren Beatty in a requisite desperate attempt to cling to lost youth.

Based on a Williams novel, this tense and foreboding film reeks of male disgust at the idea of aging sexuality. The twist here is that this can easily be interpreted as a story about aging *gay male* sexuality (Mrs. Stone is curiously called a "chicken hawk" at one point rather than a "cradle robber")—a topic too taboo for mainstream American literature and aboveground films of the time. It was perfectly acceptable, however, to denigrate the midlife female as the moribund wretch clutching at a beautiful young man, dragging him along with her toward the demise she's trying to stave off. This speaks to the fears of all men regardless of sexual orientation: aging is deadly within the male system that equates attractiveness with youth (Melamed 89). The film ends with the sinister suggestion that Mrs. Stone's empty quest to fill the "nothingness . . . the awful vacancy" (Williams 148) of her menopausal being will literally destroy her.

Leigh biographer Alexander Walker (259) called it "a brave film for Vivien to undertake," as exploring "age, abandonment, and loneliness, all her current anxieties . . . helped deflect the reality of change in her own life." Her husband, Sir Laurence Olivier, had recently divorced her for a younger woman, the ultimate salvo in an assault on her self-esteem that had begun years earlier. In 1947 she'd been eager for a role in Olivier's film version of *Hamlet*. But her beloved "Larry" thought her at thirty-four too old to play Ophelia, though he had no problem with himself at forty as Shakespeare's collegiate Dane. That "his 'age' on screen fitted the way he conceived the character" (Walker 1987, 185) made blithely convenient use of the masculine double standard; his prerogatives as the film's director let him bolster his ego further by choosing nineteen-year-old Jean Simmons as his Ophelia. Ultimately, since casting Leigh in the only other lead female role—Olivier/Hamlet's mother Gertrude—wasn't worth the risk of getting anyone's Freudian dander up, Leigh bowed out. Olivier then cast an actress six years younger than his wife to play his mother! Cinematically, this both legitimized his vision of his youthful Hamlet self and nullified the potentially formidable presence of an elder (and by male definition unattractive) woman in a sexually charged situation.

The same sexist/ageist visual dynamic was used again in 1989 by director Franco Zeffirelli in his *Hamlet*: to be seen as a sexual being deserving of her son's intrapsychic wrath, she must have the youthful appeal of a credible love interest beyond the context of the film. Zeffirelli cast Glenn Close, who'd have to have given birth to Mel Gibson's Hamlet at age nine, as Gertrude. Such forced suspension of disbelief points up a cultural maxim well served by film: what is essential is that which is attractive to the male.

Vivien Leigh's conception of herself eventually had to be "fitted" into the usual limited options for mature women, and by 1965, while starring in the stage production *La Contessa,* she was beginning to talk herself into the dubious advantages of "Sousatzka-ing" her image: "[The play is] a bridge to parts where I don't have to be a beautiful woman. . . . I thought it would make me acceptable as an actress who didn't have to be cast that way anymore" (Walker 1987, 289). One can only conjecture, albeit with reasonable certainty, where this image downshifting would ultimately have steered her career; Leigh died just two years later of a recurrence of tuberculosis.

The tradeoffs women learn to make for approval teach us to lie, then punish us for deception. From the cosmetics counter to the silver screen, we learn to objectify ourselves; to see our identities as shells as thin as the celluloid that sets the limits of our worth. But playing along means risking derision, finally, as aging hags trying to look young and not fooling anybody—which is also somehow expected of us. That Vivien Leigh's looks were reinterpreted in 1956 as a liability when Laurence Olivier deemed her "too beautiful" (Walker 1987, 228) to play his character's middle-aged wife in the stage version of *The Entertainer* (he considered having her wear a rubber mask to look the part—one wonders if it might have been green and had a wart on the end of the nose), is a damning indication of how the "average" midlife woman is perceived.

Because those who create the false images that reflect and shape our lives then blame us when the deception no longer suits them, women face a catch-22 that can only get worse with time. Even " 'powerful,' . . . 'cool,' . . . 'no-nonsense' " (Woodward 52) actresses like Glenda Jackson find fighting this system impossible: "A woman's face grows too old for films sooner than a man's" (Woodward 162). Jackson held out for as long as she could, then bit the Sousatzka bullet at forty-six to appear in *Sakarhov* (TV, 1984). "Thickly bespectacled, with her hair made into a dank grey bunch, and wearing an unflattering baggy cardigan," her biographer Ian Woodward (190) deduces, "Glenda joined the ranks of the 'non-beddable.' " "Non-beddable" was Jackson's own trenchant buzzword for the primary film devaluation of women. This aspersion denies the reality of the healthy middle-aged woman for whom intimacy, free from consequential pregnancy, may take on a new intensity. Where are our film role models for this possibility? We have yet to protest loudly enough that film, as a record of cultural history, cheats us of our heritage with a biased, one-dimensional interpretation of who we are, young and old, and especially middle-aged.

"I am now over fifty," Ellen Burstyn told *Ms.* Magazine in 1986, "not married, have one 24-year-old son, no grandchildren and, furthermore, independent and liking it" (Paige 70). How often do we get to see such women exploring their independence on film? Hollywood seems to prefer the kind of female "independence" that can be brought to justice, as in 1981's *The People vs. Jean Harris*. Burstyn starred as Harris in a video-taped courtroom docudrama "recreated in record time for a movie (TV or otherwise)" (Maltin 930)—just five weeks after Harris, fifty-six, was convicted for the killing of sixty-nine-year-old Scarsdale Diet doctor Herman Tarnower. Unusual in its reversal of male-against-female violence, this story about the female "dark side" couldn't fail to capture male attention. Harris's being a middle-aged woman who allegedly murdered a man for replacing her with a much younger rival no doubt greased the wheels on this production; it offers that most frightening of patriarchal totems: the menopausal woman who gets out of control; the Mother who can destroy. The evil old witch.

We're taught to reassure ourselves that the evil old witch brings her annihilation on herself. Children watch in relieved fascination as the Wicked Witch of the West melts away in *The Wizard of Oz* (1939); no one pays much attention to her sister of the East, who gets a house dropped on her (by a younger female) and withers under its weight. This latter image might well serve as a metaphor for the fate of the older woman in our culture. At a time when the "empty nest" (a universal symbol if not a universal reality) can weigh heavily on her sense of purpose and fulfillment, she's handed, in place of reassurance, a picture of barrenness and yearning for past glory verging on madness. She's likely to do something desperate—like kill a man.

The house in *Sunset Boulevard* (1950) belongs to the "witch," and, although she's not trapped under it, this womb symbol is no less her tomb. Gloria Swanson was ever after linked in people's minds with this classic film's Norma Desmond character, generally with an association of creaking delusion and fossilized vainglory. Swanson was in fact fifty-one when she made the film, and her Norma is no senescent caricature. The script, cowritten by director Billy Wilder and producer Charles Brackett, dredges images of the primeval destroying lover/mother from deep within the masculine unconscious in a cautionary tale about the danger of a goddess turned crone.

Norma's kinship with the sisters Wicked, East and West, is established the moment the "innocent" young hero, a starving-artist screenwriter, wanders into her silent film-era mansion like a wayward homunculus in search of incubation. He describes the place (in voiceover) as being "like that old woman in *Great Expectations*—that Miss Havisham in her rotting wedding dress and her torn veil, taking it out on the world because she'd been given the go-by." This "go-by," of course, is the penalty of male rejection, sure to turn a woman nasty even as it withers her and despite her own wealth. "A rich, powerful old maid is dangerous," Helen McNeil (72) explains the image from a literary standpoint, where, since the nineteenth century, it has stood as the scapegoat for society's anger at the unmarried elder woman who doesn't aspire to social value in selfless devotion to others. "Miss Havisham is a witch, and Dickens has her burnt alive, still wearing the white gown in which she had been abandoned at the altar decades before. Her death is, of course, her own fault."

Fame has abandoned Norma Desmond. Yet it's with the assertion of her dignity—"I *am* big. It's the pictures that got small"—that we glimpse the eternal deity whose rage at being relegated to obscurity suggests an uncanny link with the rise of patriarchal religions over "pagan" goddess consciousness.

Gutting her mystique becomes necessary from a masculine viewpoint when the young man, seduced at first by the perks her demanding needs offer, begins to fear she'll devour him. As if surrounding images of rot and funereal presentiment—rats in the empty pool; Norma's "waxworks" friends—aren't enough to warn him of his impending fate, we learn that her first husband, once a noted director, now serves as her devoted butler. Now the Pandora's box must be closed; the deadly shrine escaped; and the goddess/lover/mother's power exposed as insane delusion. Unfortunately for the young writer, hell hath no fury like—nor, perhaps, any imagemaker a worse nightmare than—an illusion scorned; Norma's bullet exacts from him the ultimate price for the unfairness of both her deification and her abandonment. Floating face-down, helpless as a dead fetus in the rejuvenated pool, he becomes a sacrifice, a life reclaimed by the great goddess at her whim. "Stars are ageless, aren't they," Norma asserts.

Like female-associated nature with its inherent capacity for destruction and inescapable push toward death, the menopausal woman becomes for men a *memento mori* figure of inevitable decline. "While not all women are affected by menopause to [an] extreme degree," gynecologist Robert A. Wilson (43) declared in his paean to estrogen therapy, *Feminine Forever,* "no woman can be sure of escaping the horror of this living decay." With "expertise" like this reflecting and perpetuating misogynist mythology, small wonder the finality of this dreadful image is tough to shake.

"[Most] of the scripts I had been offered since finishing *Sunset Boulevard* dealt with aging, eccentric actresses," Gloria Swanson wrote in 1980. "It was Hollywood's old trick: repeat a successful formula until it dies. The problem for me was that if I had played the part at a spry fifty-one, I could obviously go on playing it in its many variations for decades to come, until at last I became some sort of creepy parody of myself, or rather, of Norma Desmond—a shadow of a shadow" (Swanson 259–60).

This may prove a warning worth heeding for other actresses, like Shirley MacLaine. "Nobody knows what to do with women my age," she told *Vanity Fair* in 1991 (Collins 142). "But I am doing something about it. I've carved out this place for myself where I admit I'm fifty-six, love it, and am willing to play it." MacLaine's recent film track record belies her claim of mastery; the place she's come to, if truly of her own carving, suggests a male-identified concurrence with ignoring women her own age to focus on older, more dependably eccentric characters. More likely, she may be willing to play her actual age, but there's no place for her on the market at what Hollywood considers a "nowhere" age—too old to be "finding herself," too young to trade on the nostalgia of a bygone heyday. (Yet, ironically, she's said to have considered starring in a stage adaptation of *Sunset Boulevard* in 1987 [*Chicago Tribune* 24].) Poor Shirley's developed the warm patina of a woman who knows exactly who she is, who's acquired experience and wisdom and can give of herself from their richness. Such qualities don't address male issues of power and control, so male screenwriters aren't likely to spend much time on them.

MacLaine followed *Sousatzka* with *Steel Magnolias* (1989), playing waspish town grump Ouiser Boudreux as "66ish," exactly as specified in the original play (Harling 5). With the low-wattage "dramedy" *Waiting for the Light* (1990), she adds a daffy, ex-vaudevillian psychic auntie to her screen legacy of images of older women. Most notable for its revealing look at ageist misogyny, however, is her role in *Postcards from the Edge* (1990).

She plays Doris Mann, a glamorous, sixtyish actress/mother who on the all-important surface seems commandingly larger than life. "I'm still here!" she sings early on with the panache of a winner who indeed loves the place she's carved for herself. But later, literally stripped of her illusion, shriveled, balding, and pathetic in her hospital bed, she is revealed as a spent hag as miserable in her predicament as we are shocked at witnessing it. We're reassured that she's nothing to fear by the compassion of her daughter, the younger woman nowhere near such a fate herself yet; the figure we'd rather identify with. Doris becomes our dissociative Other: the scapegoat onto whom we can safely project an abhorrence of getting old. Then, our anxiety defused, like children for whom a switched on lamp reveals the witch in our room to be only a heap of clothing, we can watch the daughter help restore the trompe l'oeil facade; see the made-up, be-wigged Doris striding grandly off; and feel a kind of amused superiority over a pretty silly bugaboo. This is hardly a celebration of mature womanhood. Nor does it speak to us in a feminine voice.

This image doesn't exist in the novel the film was based on—Carrie Fisher's Doris is a minor background presence. The screen character is a figment of male imagination, namely that of director Mike Nichols. "Mike . . . said this mother stuff was great. People would relate to it," Fisher told *Premiere* Magazine (Green 120). Her novel was essentially thrown out in "adapting" it for film, and although Fisher did the script, "Father Mike, the cardinal of cinema" coopted her original creation and virtually commanded her to write Doris his way. "He's like the sorcerer," she remarked. "*I am the great and powerful Mike. Behind a curtain.*" He blueprinted the hospital scene and, according to Fisher, "handed me that prescription in triplicate and sent me to write [it]" (Green 120, 132).

Such arrogance underscores the bottom line in these patriarchal fantasies offered as entertainment: projecting the horror of nature's victory, unaltered by centuries of patriarchal dogma, onto nature's personification—woman. Men eschew equal rights in this area; the curse of aging is the witch's province. And as we all know, to quote Dorothy in Oz, "witches are old and ugly." The token Glenda doesn't alleviate the injustice of our being dismissed as distasteful or ignored as irrelevant at a crucial time in our lives. Those of us who even in our twenties weren't as in shape as Jane Fonda in her fifties may have trouble "loving" an age that's considered okay only if we don't look it (Melamed 130). Without a fitness obsession or the graceful legacy of dancer-trained muscles to project attractiveness, we may feel like losers with little hope of "carving out a place" for ourselves in a society that proscribes our potential. "Some women," gynecologist Wilson asserted, "when they realize [at menopause] that they are no longer women, subside into a stupor of indifference" (Wilson 44). What are we, then? And whose indifference does our scant identity on film evince?

When Madame Sousatzka proudly writes an "S" with her finger on a dusty mirror, the ephemeralness of the act underscores the transience of women's significance in a male-dominated culture and the harshness of our cinematic reflections. Film is a mirror that can lie. And since film has been effectively used to blame the female victim, it would seem that a performer like MacLaine, who delights in shucking hag makeup and in regularly pulling "ta-da!" all-glamour, all-sequined appearances at awards shows, has a certain responsibility to work toward shattering false impressions. Taking on a role that is the antithesis of what you (and other women your age) are can ultimately backfire, aiding the perpetuation of dead-end stereotypes for women. The flashy switch back to a reality far removed from the bleak illusion then becomes a reassuring performance in itself but does little to ameliorate the disservice done by the image left indelibly behind on film. It's this fictional image that's most accessible to us as an audience, that gives us a socially sanctioned pattern for our own lives as women and as such becomes a weapon of oppression—especially as we grow older. This tyranny of media and misogyny must be challenged by all of us, of course, but those whose faces become the images we relate to must use the clout that accords them *for* us, not against us. Shirley MacLaine doesn't need to bury herself under a lot of phony debris to prove she's interesting. For that matter, neither does Madame Sousatzka, who would have been no less compelling if played in her fifties to accommodate MacLaine realistically. Nor would she have lost any of her arresting personality quirks. The original title character of Bernice Rubens's novel is demanding and grandiloquent; a woman of singular style and unrequited yearning. She is also only forty-five years old.

Bette Midler was forty-six in 1991 when *For the Boys* caused preview audiences to gasp at what had "happened" to her. Her Dixie Leonard first appears as an elderly woman, a special effects eye-popper ostensibly as far from "divine" as "Miss M" might be expected to venture. But Midler's affectionate, respectful connection with Dixie communicated to viewers a credible image of a spirited individual to whom something had definitely "happened." That something, as a young minor character in the film simply summarizes, is "her life," and she wears its skin with comfortable moxie. Done in a throwback style recalling 1940s Hollywood, *For the Boys* pumps a dosage of schmaltz sufficient to cause an adverse reaction in those with a low threshold for melodrama. Yet it's in one of the film's most improbable moments that the image of the older woman is strikingly restored to timeless power.

Entertaining her son's troop in Vietnam, Dixie sees him killed in an ambush. A sequence of slow-motion visuals backed by an almost reverently poignant score leads to a pietà tableau: the grieving mother cradling her dead son. But this is not the illogically young Mary of Michelangelo's Pietà, essentially hero-worshipping a sacrificed Christ who is somehow older than she, removed from her birthgiver's claim on him, and to whom she is therefore subordinate. Dixie's son is flesh of her flesh, and while her pain presses home the intolerable reversal of parent outliving child, it also calls to mind the wise crone who has seen all, endured all, and will indeed, like nature by its eternal preeminence over what it creates, exist beyond her own offspring. This potent goddess imagery, rendering war and its unnatural destructiveness a universal mother's issue, is evoked from the moment Dixie's longtime partner Eddie tells the GIs she's there for her own boy, and for all of them as well. When, years later, she ruefully advises someone that "the thing you want to avoid is outlasting everybody," we may interpret her lament as a recognition of the dark side of the earth mother's perennial will to abide.

As with MacLaine's Sousatzka, the soul energy and projected attitude here are intimately tied to the personal connotations the role has for the actress herself—but with a notable difference. "A lot of people [thought] I must have been pretty flipped out by what I looked like," Midler commented. "But you know what? I thought I looked great. . . . I thought, if this is what I turn into, it's really not so bad." Describing Dixie as "very comforting," she embraced the character, in terms free of wreckage metaphor, as a positive possible preview of her future self: "I liked her. My husband . . . [and I decided] that we both had something to look forward to if we could be fearless. Which is hard . . . especially in our country, because people who are older get swept under the rug."

Of course, Midler had the advantage of appearing in a film that's essentially an extended flashback, so that for the most part we see her as a "younger" woman who earns her wrinkles gradually and doesn't "look like *that* for the whole picture." A superficial fearlessness, one that misses the point of Midler's application of the word, can be easily mustered in movie-makers and audiences alike when the aging process lends itself to such magical repeal. This is the allure, the function, and, for women past fair damsel days, the vengeance of the industry. Only those who, like Midler for now, can still stage a reassuring presto-change-o back to more palatable youthfulness can afford to conjure aging without sawing their appeal in half.

Movies are no different from other areas of feminist concern that, historically, have called for outspoken challengers to buck the system and establish the truth of our experience and worth as women. Hope for the future may come from insiders who, like Bette Midler, Jane Fonda, Sally Field, Goldie Hawn, Sally Kirkland, and others, have begun taking the reins behind the scenes with their own production companies; we must likewise support the efforts of women directors and writers. If they can avoid the Hollywood trap of launching projects only for younger women whose marketability is guaranteed by the same old boy-toy and baby-machine standards, we may finally have a fair legacy of women's reality on film.

A shift in perception regarding women is as vital as, and likely dependent upon, a power shift in the film industry. When, for example, Kathy Bates's menopausal Evelyn Couch laments, "I feel so useless . . . so powerless," to her new-found octogenarian friend in *Fried Green Tomatoes* (1991), we hear a familiar note, typically struck discordantly and seldom woven into a satisfying melody. But this adaptation of Fannie Flagg's 1987 novel (coscripted by Flagg and Carol Sobieski) gives us an updated tune, in our own voice, that many midlife women's lives hum realistically today. Empowerment over evanescence has hardly been a screen anthem in male renditions of female stories. Allowing this kind of noise to be made is tempting fate, jiggling the lock on that Pandora's box where years of female resentment have been accruing. Once unleashed, the accumulated force of that fury, threatening precisely because it's eminently justifiable, might drive previously "ordinary," "average" middle-aged women to aggressive revenge. In her early stages of angry realization and self-assertion, Evelyn fantasizes a kind of warrior woman/amazon goddess alter ego named Towanda to avenge her degraded Identity and jump-start her stalled potential. This persona, however lightheartedly we may relate to it, serves as an energizing transitional figure for Evelyn. When Evelyn's midlife crisis fashions her "I'm too young to be old and too old to be young" into a rallying theme and proactive epiphany, she restructures her life and thereby helps wrest images of midlife women out of negative containment. This is no small victory, given that economics determines female options on the screen much as it does in reality. Director Jon Avnet, by way of explaining why marshaling even a shoestring budget for *Fried Green Tomatoes* was tough, reasoned: "Come *on*. It's an *all*-woman movie" (Bibby 33). Obviously, even on an entertainment level, women's concerns will remain just that without equity in everything from subject matter emphasis to production decisions to public relations.

Short of such an evolution, we may be able at least to count on a demand, as the baby boomers age, for honest investigations of midlife themes, in which case both sexes will benefit from breaking free of the compulsion to defy nature; the blind spot of prizing only youth. Maybe then midlife women will be valued as individuals with full human needs, unique challenges to address and contributions to make, and healthy interests—not belittled as comic aberrations in juvenescent philosophy—in love, sex, relationships, life.

It's foolish to minimize the power of an art form which, dynamic and broadly appealing, requires nothing more than passive acceptance on our part to leave a lasting impact. As women we have always had to struggle against the socialized passivity and learned helplessness that have kept our exploration and expression of self to a dull minimum. We can't afford to acquiesce in the continued devaluation of ourselves in a medium that interprets our lives and has the potential to shape generations.

REFERENCES

Astor, Mary. 1967. *A Life on Film*. New York: Delacorte.
Barnett, Elyse Ann. 1988. "La Edad Critica: The Positive Experience of Menopause in a Small Peruvian Town." In *Women & Health: Cross-Cultural Perspectives*, compiled by Patricia Whelehan. Granby, Mass.: Bergin & Garvey.
Bibby, Bruce. February 1992. " 'Tomatoes' with Oscars." *Premiere*.
Butler, Robert N. 1985. "Psychiatry and Psychology of the Middle-Aged." In *Comprehensive Textbook of Psychiatry/IV*, 4th ed., ed. Harold I. Kaplan and Benjamin J. Sadock. Baltimore: Williams & Wilkins.
Chicago Tribune. 22 March 1991, sec. 1.
Collins, Nancy. March 1991. "The Real MacLaine." *Vanity Fair*.
Dawes, Amy. 8 August 1990. "SAG: Women Shortshrifted." *Variety*.
De Niro, Robert. 4 March 1991. Interview on CBS's "Entertainment Tonight."
Ebert, Roger. Sunday, 9 October 1988. "She Says the Strangest Things in the Most Sensible Way." *Chicago Tribune*, Arts & Show section.
Gardner, Ava. 1990. *My Story*. New York: Bantam.
Green, Jesse. November 1990. "Back from the Edge." *Premiere*.
Hackman, Gene. 7 March 1991. Interview on CBS's "Entertainment Tonight."
Harling, Robert. 1988. *Steel Magnolias*. New York: Dramatists Play Service.
MacLaine, Shirley. 16 October 1988. Interview on CBS's "Entertainment Tonight."
Maltin, Leonard (ed.). 1991. *Leonard Maltin's TV Movies and Video Guide*, 1992 ed. New York: NAL Penguin, Signet.
McNeil, Helen. 1986. *Emily Dickinson*. London: Virago.
Melamed, Elissa. 1983. *Mirror Mirror: The Terror of Not Being Young*. New York: Linden/Simon & Schuster.
Midler, Bette. 2 December 1991. Interview on ABC's "The Oprah Winfrey Show."
Miller, Jean Baker. 1976; 1986. *Toward a New Psychology of Women*. Boston: Beacon.

Paige, Connie. April 1986. "Life Is What Happens When You're Making Other Plans." *Ms*.

Seiden, Anne M. 1976. "Overview: Research on the Psychology of Women, I. Gender Differences and Sexual and Reproductive Life." *American Journal of Psychiatry* 133:9 (September): 1000.

Sjöö, Monica, and Barbara Mor. 1987. *The Great Cosmic Mother: Rediscovering the Religion of the Earth*. San Francisco: Harper & Row.

Stine, Whitney, with Bette Davis. 1974; 1975. *Mother Goddam*. New York: Hawthorn Books; New York: Berkley.

Swanson, Gloria. 1980. *Swanson on Swanson*. New York: Random House.

Variety Film Reviews, 1907–1980. 1983. Vol. 8/1949–1953. Review of *Mogambo*, *Variety*, 16 September 1953. New York: Garland.

Walker, Alexander. 1987. *Vivien: The Life of Vivien Leigh*. New York: Weidenfeld & Nicolson.

Walker, Barbara G. 1985; 1988. *The Crone: Woman of Age, Wisdom, and Power*. San Francisco, Harper & Row; Perennial Library.

Williams, Tennessee. 1950. *The Roman Spring of Mrs. Stone*. New York: New Directions.

Wilson, Robert A. 1966. *Feminine Forever*. New York: M. Evans.

Woodward, Ian. 1985. *Glenda Jackson: A Study in Fire and Ice*. New York: St. Martin's.

Meno-Boomers and Moral Guardians: An Exploration of the Cultural Construction of Menopause

Joy Webster Barbre

In a recent issue of the *Los Angeles Times,* staff writer Linda Roach Monroe asserted that the United States is about to experience a "menoboom." According to Monroe, with the aging of more than thirty million baby boom generation women, the number of women affected by menopause in the United States will increase by more than thirty-three percent over the next two decades. As the baby boomers turn into meno-boomers, menopause is likely to receive more and more of this kind of coverage in mainstream American culture. Authenticated by scientific studies and medical evidence, the information presented will probably, like Monroe's article, relate that the difficulties associated with menopause and poor health in old age may be substantially reduced when healthy living, proper medical management, and, according to some, hormone replacement therapy, begin early in the premenopausal years.

This current perspective on menopause appears to be very different from perspectives that existed in the past. For instance, one hundred years ago Victorian women were warned that menopause could cause a potpourri of ailments from shingles to insanity. And only thirty years ago our own mothers were told that, because of the "empty nest syndrome," menopause might create psychological problems. Advances in medical and scientific knowledge are often cited as the reason for these changes. While I am aware that our increased understanding of biological processes has significantly altered our ideas about menopause, I do not think that new knowledge alone can fully explain the changes. I believe we must also look at their relationship to broader cultural changes surrounding what it has meant to be a woman in the past, and what it means to be a woman today.

Menopause is a biological phenomenon with a set of physiological imperatives that do not change over time. All women who live long enough will experience or have experienced menopause. Therefore, menopause would seem to be a natural biological occurrence, over which culture has little influence. However, menopause does not occur in a vacuum. It, like other events resulting from women's reproductive biology, menstruation and childbirth for instance, is given meaning and value by the culture within which it occurs. In other words, menopause may be a biological event, but the significance attributed to it is cultural. Our perceptions of menopause are tied to the broader culture's underlying assumptions about womanhood, aging, and medicine in general. In this respect, menopause, like gender, can be seen as a cultural construct, a construct which reflects and reinforces broader cultural values and assumptions.

I contend that if we as women are to make informed decisions about the information we receive, it is important for us to recognize the culturally constructed nature of menopause. We must be aware that the model of menopause we are receiving is influenced by our culture's worldview, and we must begin to question how the advice we are offered reflects and reinforces the broader culture's underlying assumptions about women's biology, women's aging, and women's social roles in contemporary American society. In order to illustrate my point, and perhaps begin to bring into focus how the contemporary model of menopause can be seen as a cultural construct, in this essay I will explore the cultural construction of menopause in Victorian America. I have selected this period for my focus because scholars have studied the era's prescriptive literature extensively, and their work has uncovered significant links between Victorian medical advice and cultural assumptions about womanhood in nineteenth-century America (see, for example, Martin; Smith-Rosenberg; Wood).

Victorian Womanhood in America

In nineteenth-century America, the Victorian worldview was one which centered around notions of rationality, individualism, "scientific" thought, and moral authority. For the burgeoning middle class, centers of production had moved from the home to the industrial realm, and concepts of a separation between the public and private spheres were emerging. The ideal Victorian woman was perceived to be inherently intuitive, passive, delicate, affectionate, nurturing, and domestic, attributes which afforded her a dimension of moral superiority. These "innate" qualities made women unfit for the harsh and competitive realities of industrialized society (the public sphere). On the other hand, they were qualities which were best expressed in marriage and motherhood, thereby making women particularly suited to the home (private sphere). The private sphere was thus perceived as women's domain, the place where they, with their moral superiority, created an atmosphere in which men could revitalize their moral sensibilities after their exposure to corrupting immoral influences in the public sphere. The home was also the place where women's "innate" qualities could be utilized to ensure that children would be reared to responsibly fulfill their moral obligations as adults. In this manner, Victorian women came to be seen as guardians of Victorian morality.

Science, rapidly replacing religion as the realm of discourse that could best explain the universe and guide people's lives, played an important role in the rationalization and justification of these separate sphere conceptions. Though perceived as objective, and therefore the conveyor of "truth," science was in fact a part of the broader culture in which it existed. As such, it reflected and reinforced the broader culture's assumptions about how a well-ordered society should work. Medical and moral realms became intertwined as "scientific" evidence emerged which rationalized the broader culture's moral convictions, and an elaborate body of medical and biological theory explained and justified the culture's conceptions about women's inherent nature and hence their role as moral guardians (Martin; Smith-Rosenberg; Wood; Banner; Evans; Gordon; May).

Nineteenth-Century Medical Theory and Women's Bodies

Mid-nineteenth-century medical theory postulated that the ganglionic nervous system served as a storage for the "vital force" and was the source of all energy. This nervous system was directly connected to the reproductive system and the central nervous system, including the brain. This physiology was not peculiar to women, but because of women's more complex reproductive physiology—puberty, menstruation, childbirth, lactation, menopause—their reproductive organs drew more energy from the ganglionic system, and hence, their storage of "vital force" was always in danger of depletion. Any breakdown in a woman's reproductive organs could cause trauma to her nervous system and through it to other parts of her body. In a like manner, any shock to her nervous system could damage her reproductive organs. In any of these cases, extra demands were placed on her "vital forces," which were already in short supply because of her reproductive biology (Tilt). In effect, this theory rationalized what was already suspected, namely, that women and men were suited to different societal realms because of their reproductive organs.

A woman's reproductive organs governed her entire being; they dictated her personality, her abilities and limitations, and hence her social role. As Dr. Charles Meigs asserted,

> Her reproductive organs, that are peculiar to her; and in her intellect and moral perceptivity and powers, which are feminine as her organs are . . . the strange and secret influences which her organs, by their nervous constitution, and her functions, by their relation to her whole life-force, whether in sickness or health, are capable of exerting not on the body alone, but on the heart, the mind, and the very soul of woman. (38)

Dr. E. Dixon argued that reproduction was the end and object of woman's existence, the great object of her being (5, 101). Perhaps M. L. Holbrook put it most succinctly when he noted that it seemed, "as if the Almighty, in creating the female sex, had taken the Uterus and built up a woman around it" (Wood 223). Nineteenth-century medical theory meshed with moral beliefs to construct a model of female physiology that provided Victorian culture with just the kind of scientific proof it needed to explain women's inherent nature, tie women even closer to their reproductive organs, and justify the social roles ascribed to Victorian women.

With her reproductive system as the central agent for good health, the Victorian woman was admonished to lead a life that protected her ovaries and uterus. The advice given was grounded in scientific theory, but the message presented had decidedly moral overtones, and the imperatives for a healthy life were ones which reinforced Victorian conceptions about women's social roles. Employment; social activism; contraception; excesses in food, dress, or sexuality; novel reading; and education were all activities that could over-stimulate a woman's nervous system and thus endanger her reproductive system. Further, birth control was risky because it prevented semen from "bathing the female reproductive organs," an act which neutralized the excessive nervous stimulation built up during sexual excitement. At the same time, excess sexual activity was dangerous because it created nervous exhaustion, thereby depleting the energy sources to the reproductive system (Smith-Rosenberg and Rosenberg 14–19).

In a like manner, education presented particular peril because it diverted the "vital force" away from the uterus, and to the brain. As one respected doctor reported,

> I have known many to lose their catamenia [menstruation] by severe application of the mind to studies . . . to rack her brain learning Latin is nonsense. She can't learn it, in the first place. She can only try till it makes her sick . . . they [women] cannot . . . participate in the affairs of nations or municipalities, because by the very nature of their moral and physical constitution, they are bound to the horns of the family altar . . . the only arithmetical calculation she requires is the relation between one dozen eggs at 12½ cents and three dozen at the same rate. . . . (Meigs 352–64)

Clearly, nineteenth-century conceptions about women's biology were tightly bound to the ideology surrounding women's social roles and promoted woman's position as moral guardian. And when Victorian assumptions about women's aging are also explored, we can begin to see how the era's construction of womanhood shaped the meanings and values ascribed to menopause during this period.

Definitions of Female Old Age in
Victorian America

During the nineteenth century, when the uterus was the primary definer of womanhood and menopause signaled the end of the very core of woman's existence, menopause heralded the onset of female old age. (Prior to this period, old age for women was perceived to begin at about 60 years of age; see, for example, Demos; Premo.) The very title of Dr. E. J. Tilt's influential nineteenth-century book indicates his stand on the issue: *The Change of Life . . . Women at the Decline of Life.* In his preface, Tilt reported that he was about to " . . . describe the closing scenes of the life of women" (6). Another doctor described menopause as the "climax of life-force . . . the possessor to decline toward the last term of existence . . . she has now become an old woman . . . " (Meigs 444). And yet another referred to menopause as " . . . a transition to the closing phase of her existence" (Dixon 101). By mid-nineteenth century, many women were living well into old age. In 1870 the average life span for women was about sixty-five, women over sixty-five made up three percent of the total population, and one half of those over sixty-five were women (see, for example, Achenbaum 91–92; Fisher 279; Premo 16). Victorian doctors set the average age for menopause at forty-five (Tilt 21; Meigs 453). Thus, while large numbers of nineteenth-century women had many years of life left after menopause, the culture considered them years of old age.

In Victorian culture female old age was often presented as a pleasurable stage of life. Many doctors asserted that, with the debilitating effects of menstruation and childbearing behind them, postmenopausal women not only regained the beauty and health of their younger days, but in fact those qualities were enhanced by the plumpness that resulted from menopause (Meigs 445; Tilt 103–105). In addition, because older people were thought to have discovered the code of behavior that ensured a long life, old age was romanticized in the second half of the nineteenth century. As historian Andrew Achenbaum has noted, "Precisely because most Americans believed that one's mental outlook and personal habits affected chances for living a full life, older men and women . . . demonstrated which lifestyles were more effective than others for promoting healthful longevity" (15). Old women, possessing the natural moral endowment of their sex and the acquired status of an exemplary long life, were doubly romanticized (Achenbaum).

This romanticization is clearly evident in the medical literature. Tilt noted that once menopause had passed,

> love still rules paramount in the breast of women, . . . it still engrosses the thoughts, . . . crowning the evening of life with unanticipated happiness. . . . becoming the guides, the supports and the mainstays of both sexes in the difficulties of life. Indeed, it would not be too much to say that the discordant elements of society can never be blended without the authority willingly conceded to the combined influence of age and sex. (103)

Dixon wrote, "The crowning glory of a healthy woman is a large family . . . when faithfully carried out . . . she is adding to her length of years, and the happiness of her old age" (315).

Ideally, for the postmenopausal Victorian woman life was to be a continuation of the nurturing, domestic, and moral aspects of her younger days, but with the added dimensions of improved health and beauty and veneration and respect for her example of right living. Women could enjoy the promise of old age, but not until they had passed through menopause, a period of danger laden with physical risks and hidden cultural significance.

Victorian Perceptions of Menopause

Menopause was the point at which the system that had regulated women's entire lives failed, and the crisis it presented was not to be taken lightly. Doctors asserted that because of the integral connection between women's reproductive organs and their central nervous systems, menopause, when the reproductive organs were in a disturbed state, " . . . is universally admitted to be a critical and dangerous time for her" (Tilt 15). Chronic ill health, chronic debility, consumption, rheumatism, ulcerated legs, diabetes, urinary tract problems, hemorrhoids, gout, tooth decay, heart disease, shingles, chronic diarrhea and constipation, deafness, and cancer are just a few of the conditions doctors warned could be brought on by menopause (Tilt 106–224).

Reflecting the culture's emphasis on women's moral superiority, one of the most serious conditions associated with menopause was "moral insanity." E. J. Tilt explained "moral insanity" by noting that

> During the change of life the nervous system is so unhinged that the management of the mental and moral faculties often taxes the ingenuity of the medical confidant . . . [the disturbance] can cause normally moral women to act without principle . . . be untruthful . . . be peevish . . . even have fits of temper . . . steal . . . leave their families . . . brood in melancholy self absorption. (1882, 101)

The perceived association between menopause and moral insanity was so pervasive that Victorian era court records indicate moral insanity due to menopause was often accepted as a defense in cases of shoplifting (Abelson 184–87). While the ailments listed above were perceived to be the result of menopause, prescriptions for surviving this dangerous period of life indicate that a woman's behavior determined whether she would have the kind of menopause that caused these conditions.

Packaged as medical advice, the counsel about menopause given to Victorian women stressed the critical nature of the experience, but it also conveyed a warning that the hazards of menopause could be avoided if women held fast to their "innate" nurturing, delicate, and moral nature. The morally questionable acts of novel reading, sexual intercourse, dancing, going to the theater or parties, and displays of temper were all risky because they excited the nervous system and hence endangered the reproductive organs (Tilt 48, 73, 94–99; Meigs 464). Emphasizing the delicate and fragile nature of women, most doctors prescribed a quiet life at this time. Tilt recommended long periods of rest and the avoidance of any

kind of excitement during this period (189). Dixon wrote, "The first caution we would urge upon the female relates to . . . the management of her
temper . . . the mind and the uterine system should remain in profound
repose" (105, 108). Another advised, " . . . keep the mind not stupefied,
certainly, but in a calm and complacent mood" (Meigs 369). In essence,
women were advised to retire from the world, devote themselves to do-
mesticity, and concentrate on their roles as moral guardians.

For the nineteenth-century woman, it was not only her behavior during
menopause that determined the kind of old age she would have; the accumulated experiences of her past life were also a contributing factor. Indis-
cretions in earlier life, as one doctor noted, " . . . will find this period
[menopause] a veritable Pandora's box of ills" (Haller 65). Dr. J. H. Kellogg asserted that " . . . the grey haired women who have passed their
climacteric, who frequent the offices of popular gynecologists . . . are to a
large extent victims of sexual transgressions." He also argued that birth
control and abortion were, " . . . injurious to character and led to the
most wretched diseases in women's later years" (350). Mrs. Emma Drake,
M.D., advised that women who ignored their physical nature would pay
the consequences at menopause. The detrimental effects of dancing, exercise, improper dress, and education might not be felt until menopause but,
" . . . at the crisis, when a reserve force is needed, they find themselves
without it, and go down with the current to days of suffering, if not death
itself." On birth control and abortion Drake warned,

> Women who have lent their souls to this heartless work, will, if they per-
> sist, go to swell the number of those who suffer not only discomfort, but
> disease and lifelong suffering at the time and after the menopause. Nature
> has become so outraged that she can never again adjust the proper working
> of the physical system. (131)

Charles Meigs asserted that " . . . a badly passed youth will show up in a
disastrous menopause," and related the example of a young woman who
attempted to delay the onset of her monthly menses by cold baths so that
she might attend a dance. Meigs reported that her efforts were successful,
but at the change of life she suffered diseases of the womb which were
directly related to this one incident (349–55). A young girl's decision to
neglect the imperatives of her biology in favor of the morally questionable
act of dancing doomed her to problems during her menopausal years. In
effect, menopause and its signaling of old age became an event of moral
reckoning for Victorian women.

For nineteenth-century Victorian women, representations of old age

held the promise of comfortable fulfillment and familial and societal reverence. But the prelude to old age, menopause, was fraught with danger, the
point at which previous violations of their moral and delicate nature took
their toll. The prescriptive model for surviving those dangers and receiving
the rewards of old age was a model based on "objective" scientific evidence, but one that was also decidedly in tune with the definition of womanhood in Victorian America. It was a model which stressed and
reinforced the delicate, nurturing, and moral qualities assumed to be a
part of Victorian womanhood, whether or not the essential element of
reproductive capability was present.

Women, Culture, and Menopause in Contemporary America

Today's model of womanhood appears to bear little resemblance to the
nineteenth-century model described above. Reproduction is still a core element in our culture's definition of woman, but giving birth and rearing
children comprise only one option in a woman's life, not the very reason
for her existence. For modern woman a whole spectrum of choices, experiences, and social roles are available. And yet, it is impossible to open a
magazine, watch a television show, or view a movie without receiving our
culture's definition of ideal womanhood. No matter what the choices, or
age, today's woman is competent and capable in all areas. She is able to
succeed in her chosen career, raise perfect children, create the perfect
home, and juggle the numerous demands of all three. She is sexually re-
sponsive, youthfully attractive, intellectually stimulated, and thus a perfect
companion for the man in her life. She keeps up on current affairs, supports
the right causes, and knows what foods and behaviors are scientifically
proven to be best for the human body. In her busy schedule she finds time
to take care of herself in order to assure that she will be attractive, energetic, physically fit, and healthy well into old age. On this model of womanhood the menopausal woman differs little from her younger sister. Images
that reflect the ideal woman smile out at us from the covers of *Lears* magazine, and Jane Fonda is admired as the exemplary menopausal woman.

However, like our Victorian sisters a century ago, we, the women of
today, are also warned that menopause is a crisis. As Dr. Wulf H. Utian
recently wrote,

> Many women perceive menopause—like menses and pregnancy—as just
> another physiologic event in the course of female reproduction, and do not

seek medical help. . . . We now know that menopausal symptoms must not be ignored. Even 'asymptomatic menopause' may initiate silent, progressive, and ultimately lethal sequelae. (2)

The definition of "sequelae" is "a pathological condition resulting from a disease" (*American Heritage Dictionary* 1982). The disease in question here is estrogen deficiency disease, a disease which, we are warned, causes pathological conditions. The cause of this disease is reported to be menopause.

According to numerous medical and scientific experts and commercial drug companies, hormone replacement therapy (HRT) is an important treatment for this disease, and many advise that women begin a program of HRT at or before menopause and continue therapy for the rest of their lives. "The American College of Obstetrics and Gynecology recommends that every woman be considered for HRT . . . " (Monroe 1). Echoing the sentiments of the majority of this association's conferees at a recent conference on menopause, one speaker stated, "It is becoming increasingly clear that estrogen therapy has an important second purpose, that is, prevention of disease. This second aspect of estrogen therapy should prompt serious consideration of estrogen replacement therapy for every woman at the time of menopause" (Ettinger 1298). And Robert G. Wells, M.D., director of The Menopause Center, recently wrote, "With so many benefits and virtually no dangers, it now seems reasonable to recommend that all post-menopausal women—regardless of age or menopausal symptoms—seriously be considered for hormone replacement therapy" (67).

The assertion that HRT is a reasonable course of treatment for all women is not new. Roughly thirty years ago, when our mothers were being told that the "empty nest syndrome" could cause psychological problems at menopause, Dr. Robert Wilson wrote his best seller, *Feminine Forever,* in which he asserted that, with HRT, "Menopause is curable . . . Menopause is completely preventable . . . Instead of being condemned to witness the death of their own womanhood . . . [women] will remain fully feminine—physically and emotionally—for as long as they live" (15–19). In the 1990s, Wilson's rationale for advocating HRT seems chauvinistic and even anachronistic. Few of us view menopause as the death of womanhood. And yet, at that time, on the prevailing model of womanhood as represented by June Cleaver, Donna Reed, and Margaret Anderson, femininity was virtually synonymous with motherhood. Wilson's medical advice was shaped and formed by the culture's assumption that menopause presented a psychological crisis in women's lives and, like the Victorian doctors before him, his underlying message reflected and reinforced the era's cultural assumptions about women's social roles and women's biology.

Contemporary proponents of HRT have drawn their conclusions from the evidence provided by "objective" scientific studies. We must remember, however, that today, as in the 1960s and the nineteenth century, science does not stand outside of culture; it is a part of the culture in which it exists, and therefore "objectivity" is, at best, a nebulous term. Scientific evidence in the nineteenth century "proved" that menopause was a physiological crisis with moral overtones. In the early 1960s, scientific thought proposed that HRT could circumvent the psychological crisis menopause caused in women's sense of femininity. Today the scientific evidence once again suggests that menopause is a physiological crisis; but as in the 1960s and the nineteenth century, the unspoken message reinforces and reflects our current model of ideal womanhood. For instance, as previously noted, today's ideal woman, whatever her age, is youthfully attractive and physically fit. Robert G. Wells recently wrote, "HRT may not be the elusive 'fountain of youth,' but is surely qualifies as one of its 'springs' " (70). This claim for the benefits of HRT may provide us with a starting point in our search for the ways in which current advice on menopause constructs a model of menopause which is consistent with contemporary cultural assumptions about women's biology, women's social roles, and women's aging.

Definitions of what it means to be a woman have been constructed in different ways at different times throughout America's history. These changing definitions have emerged from changing broader cultural assumptions about how the world works. However, one essential element in all of these definitions has remained constant—woman's physiological ability to reproduce. And yet, the natural biological process of menopause—the end of those reproductive abilities—is an unavoidable experience for most women. It is an event which all definitions of womanhood must somehow accommodate in ways that are consistent with broader definitions of womanhood. Just as the models presented to women in the past must be questioned for the ways in which they were constructed to accomplish this accommodation, we, the women of today, must also question the model we are receiving. We must ask if the current rush to save us from menopause is the result of new "objective" medical and scientific knowledge—a breakthrough in human's ability to correct nature's mistakes. Or is the perceived need to save women influenced by something more complex—specifically, by current assumptions about women's biology, women's social roles, and women's aging, as well as the broader cultural values that prevail in America today?

REFERENCES

Abelson, Elaine S. 1989. *When Ladies Go A-Thieving: Middle-Class Shoplifters in the Victorian Department Store*. New York: Oxford University Press.
Achenbaum, W. Andrew. 1978. *Old Age in the New Land: The American Experience Since 1790*. Baltimore: Johns Hopkins University Press.
American Heritage Dictionary, 2nd College Edition. 1982. Boston: Houghton Mifflin.
Banner, Lois W. 1983. *American Beauty*. Chicago: University of Chicago Press.
Demos, John. 1983. "Old Age in Early New England." *The American Family in Social-Historical Perspective*. Ed. Michael Gordon. New York: St. Martin's.
Dixon, Edward Henry, M.D. 1857. *Woman and Her Diseases, from the Cradle to the Grave*. New York: A. Ranney.
Drake, Mrs. Emma F. Angell, M.D. 1902. *What a Woman of Forty-Five Ought to Know*. London: Vir.
Ettinger, Bruce, M.D. May 1987. "Overview of the Efficacy of Hormonal Replacement Therapy." *American Journal of Obstetrics and Gynecology*. 1298.
Evans, Sara M. 1989. *Born for Liberty: A History of Women in America*. New York: The Free Press.
Fisher, David Hackett. 1978. *Growing Old in America*. New York: Oxford University Press.
Gordon, Linda. 1977. *Woman's Body, Woman's Right*. New York: Penguin.
Haller, John S., Jr. 1972. "From Maidenhood to Menopause: Sex Education for Women in Victorian America." *Journal of Popular Culture* 6, no. 1. 49–70.
Kellogg, J. H., M.D. 1893. *Ladies Guide in Health and Disease*. Battle Creek, Mich.: Modern Medicine.
Martin, Emily. 1987. *The Woman in the Body: A Cultural Analysis of Reproduction*. Boston: Beacon.
May, Elaine Tyler. 1980. *Great Expectations: Marriage & Divorce in Post-Victorian America*. Chicago: University of Chicago Press.
Meigs, Charles. 1848. *Females and Their Diseases*. Philadelphia: Lea and Blanchard.
Monroe, Linda Roach. 5 December 1989. "Menopause: Baby Boomers' Next Step." *Los Angeles Times*, E. 1–3.
Premo, Terri L. 1983. "Women Growing Old in the New Republic: Personal Responses to Old Age, 1785–1835." Diss. University of Cincinnati.
Smith-Rosenberg, Carroll. 1973. "Puberty to Menopause: The Cycle of Femininity in Nineteenth Century America." *Feminist Studies* 1, no. 3/4. 58–72.
Smith-Rosenberg, Carroll, and Charles Rosenberg. 1984. "The Female Animal." *Women and Health in America*. Ed. Judith Walzer Leavitt. Madison: University of Wisconsin Press.
Tilt, Edward John, M.D. 1882. *The Change of Life in Health and Disease. A Clinical Treatise on the Diseases of the Ganglionic Nervous System Incidental to Women at the Decline of Life*. 4th Ed. New York: Bermingham.

Utian, Wulf H., M.D. 1989. "Renewing Our Commitment to the Remaining 85%." *Menopause Management* 2, no. 1. 2.
Wells, Robert G., M.D. 1989. "Should All Postmenopausal Women Receive Hormone Replacement Therapy?" *Senior Patient* 6, no. 1. 65–70.
Wilson, Robert A., M.D. 1966. *Feminine Forever.* New York: M. Evans.
Wood, Ann Douglas. 1984. "The Fashionable Diseases: Women's Complaints and Their Treatment in Nineteenth Century America." *Women and Health in America.* Ed. Judith Walzer Leavitt. Madison: University of Wisconsin Press.

Metaphors of Menopause: The Metalanguage of Menopause Research

Geri L. Dickson

What types of knowledge do you want to disqualify in the very instance of your demand: "Is it a science?" Which speaking, discoursing subjects—which subjects of experience and knowledge—do you then want to "diminish" when you say: "I who conduct this discourse am conducting a scientific discourse, and I am a scientist?"

—*Foucault*

Our conceptual systems, in terms of thought, language, and action, are metaphoric in nature. Metaphors, according to Lakoff and Johnson, are related to facts and are capable of containing and transmitting knowledge; they have genuine meaning. Because metaphors are bits of language that imply a relationship of similarity between two things, they reflect beliefs and convey attitudes. The study of the metaphors used to describe or express a phenomenon in language is a way of shedding new light on that phenomenon.

The language of the scientific discourses and practices of the Western world have contributed to the evolution of a picture of the menopausal woman as irritable, frequently depressed, tired, asexual, and overwhelmed by hot flashes. These stereotypes of midlife women impose restricted positions on women as they are classified as products of their reproductive systems and their hormones. The available research on midlife women, most often conceptualized from a biomedical perspective, studies menopause as a "hormone deficiency disease": a cluster of symptoms, led by hot flashes and vaginal atrophy, including, also, many diffuse psychological problems. Little research data are available that have not been strongly filtered through the biomedical perspective.

Menopause, simply put, is the cessation of menses that without pathology or medical intervention occurs around the fiftieth birthday of women. The last menstrual flow represents a marker in the transition from a reproductive state to a nonreproductive state. Although menopause is a universal and definitive landmark of aging, knowledge generated from cross-cultural studies suggests that women of different cultures experience the menopausal transition in different ways (Beyene; Flint 1982; Lock).

The discourse of science, according to Popkewitz, can be viewed as having different layers of abstraction. These layers exist simultaneously and are superimposed one upon another. At one level, the language of science focuses on the question, the content, and the procedures of research. However, at a deeper, paradigmatic level we can view inquiry as metalanguage in which the narrative creates a particular style or form for thought. As Popkewitz explains, "The metalanguage maintains assumptions which are unconscious in the formal debates of science but by which the content and procedures of inquiry are made sensible and plausible" (33). Within the discourses, science's very language builds certain images of social reality through the words and rules of the language. This scientific language is never neutral but is filled with conscious and unconscious assumptions about both what the world is like and the nature of things. As an exemplar of the human construction of scientific inquiry, the study of women and menopause provides evidence to illuminate the social connection between science and societal values that combine to assign aging women to a maligned and marginal status in our society (McCrea).

The focus of study reported here was an exploration of the interrelationship among the underlying assumptions about science and about women, and the conceptualizations of menopause in the discourses of differing paradigms of research. Four scientific paradigms of menopausal research, with differing foundational assumptions, were identified: the biomedical, the sociocultural, a feminist, and a postmodern. A philosophical analysis of the metalanguage of the four paradigms, using selected exemplars of each paradigm, illuminates and clarifies the links between the research assumptions and their theoretical perspectives of menopause. A discussion is presented of the differing research paradigms, beliefs and assumptions, conceptualizations and metaphors of menopause found in the language of research.

The Biomedical Paradigm

The groundwork for the current conceptualization of menopause as a disease began with hormone studies in the 1930s and 1940s. According to Bell, it was believed that the form, function, and behavior of females could be demonstrated in a dispassionately empirical way, thereby attributing the cause of women's behavior to biological processes. The traditional scientific method, based on the use of controls, correlation of data obtained by different observers, and the collection and quantification of large numbers of observations, raised the possibility of treating, as a disease, the decrease in hormones in women at midlife (Bell).

Three crucial sets of assumptions can be teased from the metalanguage of biomedical menopause research using a Kuhnian paradigm analysis. They can be summarized as: (a) science is empirical validation that results in true knowledge; it is objective and value-free, and is based on a linear, causal model; (b) women are primarily products of their reproductive systems and hormones; and (c) there is something inherently pathological in the female's reproductive system (Dickson 1990a, 1990b). Based on these three sets of assumptions, overlaid one on top of another, menopause is studied as biomedical variables, treatments, and outcomes.

Underlying Assumptions about Science. The criteria for evaluating knowledge in the biomedical paradigm are based upon assumptions of science as an objective, precise, rigorous search for the relationship between facts of an ordered reality in which law-like regularities can be identified, tested, and verified (Dickson, 1989; Voda and George; H. S. Wilson). This worldview of science is based on empiricism and has been identified by some as the empirical/analytical paradigm of science (Allen et al.; Morgan; Popkewitz).

Cook described the basic assumptions of the empirical/analytical paradigm as "built on the supposition that an external world of objects exists, that these objects are lawfully interrelated, and that the relationships are mediated by a real force in objects that is called causation" (78). The basic aims of science have been identified by Kerlinger as explanation, prediction, and control; theory development is the ultimate aim. The adequacy of a theory can be judged by its predictive power, that is, its ability to state, under certain conditions, a relationship between one class of empirical events and another (Kerlinger).

The purpose of scientific studies has been identified by Cook as the probing of "causal relations between manipulated independent variables (treatments) and measured outcomes" (74). To manipulate variables and measure outcomes, it is necessary to control such things as the environment, conditions, subjects, and treatment. In menopause studies, for example, a focus has developed on experimental studies that relate the effects of hormone replacement therapy (treatment) to the prevention of osteoporosis (outcome) (Genant et al.; Lindsay et al.; Riggs et al. 1986), and more recently to heart disease (Barrett-Connor).

Underlying Assumptions about Women. The assumptions about women arise from the Freudian belief that biology is destiny and women are assumed to be "the 'victims' of their changing bodies and fluctuating hormones" (Voda and George 56). The functions of women are determined biologically, and when reproduction is no longer possible, women are considered medically old and socially useless (Cohen). Accompanying this view is the belief that the physiological changes of menopause result in increased psychological distress (Lennon 1987).

As Zita in her essay in this volume points out, an example of the biomedical view of women and menopause can be found in a report of work on hormone replacement therapy published in a peer-reviewed medical journal. Wilson and Wilson wrote: "The unpalatable truth must be faced that all postmenopausal women are castrates. . . . Our streets abound with them—walking stiffly in twos and threes, seeing little and observing less. It is not unusual to see an erect man of 75 vigorously striding along on a golf course, but never a woman of this age (362)." At first glance, this may appear to be an outdated view of women, but the male continues as the norm of the aging process. Therefore, the assumption of the "abnormal" nature of older women continues to be reinforced (Cohen; Fausto-Sterling).

Conceptualization of Menopause. The assumptions about the reality of menopause flow from the belief that the menopausal transition is a hormone deficiency disease, similar to diabetes, and treatable with hormone replacement therapy (Henig). The social and the scientific have coalesced to support the goal, advocated by physician-researcher Nachtigall, of preventing aging in women by returning women to their premenopausal physiological states with the use of hormones: the question is not raised as to who will benefit—women or the drug companies—if women return to their premenopausal physiological states.

Existing evidence indicates that the current state-of-the-art of biomedical research is based on data from a relatively small proportion of self-selecting women who experience and report problems, utilize health facilities, and are, therefore, conveniently available as research subjects (McKinlay and McKinlay; Voda and George). The knowledge generated from these convenience-sample studies of predominantly patient populations is a clinical stereotype of the "typical" menopausal woman who presents a broad range of often diffuse symptoms and, consequently, consumes a disproportionate share of health resources (McKinlay et al.).

Further, very little data have been collected about the normal range of menopause experiences. In a comprehensive review of menopause studies,

McKinlay and McKinlay reported that scarce data were available about the normal menopause; Delaney et al. reported that little has changed, since the 1970s, regarding available data.

Metaphors of Menopause in the Language of Biomedical Research. The specific historical base for the biomedical discourses and metaphors was laid in the nineteenth century with the medicalization of women's bodies: normal reproductive functions were treated as diseases. Foucault (1980), in his studies of sexuality, described how the female body was analyzed from the nineteenth century onward "as being thoroughly saturated with sexuality, whereby it was integrated into the sphere of medical practices, by reason of a pathology intrinsic to it" (104). The specter of the nineteenth-century science that was able to provide a plausible account of the sexual origins of the inferiority of women (Russett) was later found in the work of Deutsch.

Deutsch, a student of Freud, presented a view of motherhood and womanhood as one and the same in which the menopausal years became a struggle against the inevitable disaster of the physiological process of aging. Subsequent researchers built upon Deutsch's case studies of her psychiatric patients and carried forward her assumptions about women and menopause (McKinlay and McKinlay; Voda and George). In addition, there often is a strongly held belief in this kind of research that the individual woman is responsible for her own problematic experiences in menopause: "the prognosis for an uncomplicated, mildly disturbing menopause and climacteric is excellent for the *well-adjusted, informed* woman" [italics added] (Iatrakis et al., 117).

The language of the knowledge of menopause in the biomedical literature provides images of menopause as a breakdown of central control and failed production (Martin). Menopause is depicted by metaphors of disease or abnormal degeneration such as found in the following examples: "sex-steroid deficiency" (Riggs and Melton), "estrogen withdrawal symptoms (Ravnikar), "loss of femininity" (Lennon 1982), "vegetative symptomatology" (Berg and Hammar), and "problems that need estrogen replacement therapy" (Ferguson et al.).

Outcomes of this type of research indicate that the failure of female reproductive organs to produce estrogen after menopause is debilitating to health and leads to other diseases, such as osteoporosis (Martin) and, more recently, cardiovascular disease (Barrett-Connor). In addition, viewed from a different paradigmatic perspective, these experimental studies can be seen to limit and exclude the possibilities of alternative solutions for the prevention of osteoporosis or heart disease. The biomedical approach, with its paradigmatic assumptions and methodologies, lays "the ground work for hormone replacement therapy as a logical and 'scientific' choice to prevent and treat osteoporosis" (MacPherson 1985, 11) or heart disease.

The Sociocultural Paradigm

In response to this ideology of the biomedical view and its negative implications for women, a second paradigm evolved in the 1970s, based on differing assumptions about science, about women, and about menopause. This literature remains a competing body of knowledge, but it contains a much smaller number of studies than that within the biomedical paradigm.

Underlying Assumptions about Science. Although the methods of research may vary, the epistemology of the sociocultural paradigm arises from assumptions about science that are similar to those in the empirical/analytical paradigm: here science also is based on a linear, causal model (Voda and George). However, the cause of any problem is social or cultural, rather than biological.

The assumptions about the world in the sociocultural view begin with a belief in the nature of the world as more dynamic than it is thought to be according to the assumptions underlying the biomedical approach. Experimental or quasi-experimental design studies are not usually conducted within this paradigm. The everyday-life world is important; research is conducted in field, not laboratory, studies. The actions of people are not considered the "facts" of science; rather, attention is given to the attitudes, relationships, roles, and interactions in a particular society and/or culture (Leininger; Wilson). The variables of interest are social and cultural in origin, and the assumption is embraced that it is the position of women and societal conditions that contribute to the reactions of women to menopause (McCrea; Posner; Voda and George).

Assumptions about the purpose of sociocultural menopause research, suggested by Lock, include: "investigat[ing] the meaning of the social transitions under study for the individual informant, in the context of her personal life history, social roles, and particular culture" (23). The roots and effects of knowledge and power, rather than being vested in the scientific discourse and clinical jurisprudence, as in the biomedical paradigm, are found in the everyday language of cultural, social, environmental, and philosophical phenomena.

Underlying Assumptions about Women. No longer are women viewed as being at the mercy of their fluctuating hormones or their biology. It is assumed, instead, that there is "no consistent relationship between the biochemical or physiological changes and behaviors" (Voda and George 61). By opting for the sociocultural approach, an attempt is made to discredit the assumption of the biomedical approach that women are physically and emotionally handicapped by menstruation and menopause.

Conceptualization of Menopause. Menopause is viewed as a natural process through which most women pass with minimum difficulty, not a disease process (McCrea). Kaufert (1982) stressed that menopause is a culturally constructed event to which people bring preconceived ideas about its nature. Contesting the biomedical assumption that menopause is a hormone deficiency disease, researchers within this paradigm often study cultures where women do not experience the same kinds of responses to menopause that women in the United States seem to experience. Their assumption is that true physiological variants of menopause are present in all women, not just in the modern Western population (Beyene).

Metaphors of Menopause in the Language of Sociocultural Research. The metaphors of menopause in the language of the sociocultural research differ from those in the biomedical studies. The "experience of menopause" or the "response to menopause" is the terminology used, rather than the distancing language referring to "the menopause," as often found in the biomedical paradigm. Metaphors of menopause include: "a developmental phase" (Hotchner); "a developmental event precipitated by the aging processes of the endocrine system" (Uphold and Susman 1985); "a natural stage, a transitional phase in a woman's life" (Frey); "a period of life" (Polit and LaRocco); and "alterations in wellness" (Engel). Other locutions from a cultural perspective include: "cultural construction" (Lock); "culturally constructed event" (Kaufert 1982); "preconceived ideas about its nature" (Kaufert 1986); "psychological and cultural artifacts" (Walfisch et al.); "midlife conflict" (Goldstein); and "cultural context which shapes the pattern of a woman's roles" (Beyene). The conceptualization, images, and metaphors of menopause in the sociocultural approach are more varied than those found in the biomedical paradigm.

The historical basis for the sociocultural paradigm can be found in the work of Flint (1975). From her research, Flint concluded that the difference between the two million women in the United States with severe symptoms and the absence of incapacitation of Indian women during menopause could be attributed to differences in the attitudes the two cultures exhibit toward menopausal women. In the Indian culture, older women experience a heightened social prestige, whereas "in our culture, there is no reward for attaining menopause" (Flint 1975, 163). A comprehensive review of cultural menopausal research by Wilbush (1982) added support to the view of menopausal symptomatology as a phenomenon of Western cultural behavior.

In addition to the cultural studies on women's reactions to menopause, social studies have been conducted in an attempt to link reactions to menopause with social roles. A foundational assumption of these studies is "that women experience reactions to the [menopausal transition] that are unpleasant and that these are rooted in the quantity and quality of social roles and relationships in their lives" (Voda and George 67). The childrearing role and the marital role (Dosey and Dosey; Uphold and Susman 1981), as well as the work role (Polit and LaRocco; Uphold and Susman 1985), were the emphasis of studies to determine the relationship between any unpleasant reactions to the transition and the various roles of women.

A Feminist Paradigm

Underlying Assumptions. Feminist theory and research covers a broad spectrum of writings and feminist science presumes and utilizes a variety of assumptions and methods (Harding). Nevertheless, the underlying assumptions of feminist studies revolve around a view of the world as a place in which men have defined what being a woman means in the larger society. The studies presented are in the nature of a critique that exposes social conditions that hinder human communication and liberation (Bell; McCrea; MacPherson 1981, 1985). Feminists have sought to develop a new paradigm of social criticism that does not rely on traditional philosophical assumptions (Nicholson). Thus, feminist science often takes the form of an emancipatory sociocultural critique.

From this perspective, the entire tradition of Western science is challenged by exposing how the foundations of knowledge have been built on the assumptions of male domination and patriarchal power (Fee). The assumption is that "social life is structured by meaning, by rules, conventions, or habits adhered to by individuals as social beings" (Allen et al., 34). The aim of this research is the possibility of gaining an understanding of the patterns that structure human activity by exposing the relationship between the meanings of human activity and existing social structures. Feminists concentrate on the social and political forces found in the domination of women.

The number of feminist studies of menopause is small, and most of them are on the menstrual cycle. Posner speculated that the dearth of feminist literature on menopause resulted from a move away from doing research that focused on cyclical changes in women. However, Bleier and Harding have argued that cultural prejudices often have been disguised as scientific facts founded in a belief that women are physically and emotionally handicapped by the menstrual cycle and therefore are subordinate to men. In addition, as Whatley and others have indicated, traditional definitions of female bodies, health, and sexuality have been constructed and defined in male terms. Therefore, the uniqueness of "womanhood" often has been limited to menstruation and, of interest here, menopause. This thinking continues to perpetuate the social ideology of women as sex objects and reproductive organs (McCrea) and can be used to limit social possibilities for women (Delaney et al.).

Underlying Assumptions about Women. A foundational assumption in feminist menopause research is that women are not defined by their hormones. However, there is sometimes a tendency to develop essentialist assumptions about the nature of human beings (that there is an essential feminine or masculine nature) and the conditions for social life (Nicholson). Thus, in criticizing the feminist theories that underlie feminist research, Weedon points out that these theories often espouse the view that "there is an essential womanhood, common to all women, suppressed or repressed by patriarchy" (10). Not only does this drift toward essentialism undermine the feminist insight that conceptual construction accounts for the traditional, patriarchal conceptualization of the essential nature of women; it leads some theorists into a fault that is the mirror image of the patriarchal mistake. That is, in attempting to overcome the oppressive assumptions about women embedded in the traditional approaches, some feminist theorists have posited what they take to be (essentially) a feminine perspective, utilized that perspective to define "woman," and then taken woman so defined as the norm, with man as "the other." Building research on such universalist and normative assumptions leaves little room to explore and identify what may be the very different experiences of women of different cultures, classes, and colors.

Conceptualization of Menopause. The conceptualization of menopause in the feminist literature is as a natural female process with social and often class implications. Menopause is envisioned as a tabooed subject, veiled in secrecy and silence, in which women's rights are suppressed in the name of biology (Delaney et al.; MacPherson 1981, 1985; Weideger). The suppression of women's positions in the name of biology has led to the social control of women through the medicalization of menopause.

MacPherson (1981) clearly documented how the medical community has responded with "treatments" for women that helped to create the submissive female patient. Further, according to MacPherson (1981), "this disease model has been socially constructed during the past 150 years by science, medicine, government, and the drug industry to gain power, profits, and social control over women" (100). With the transformation of menopause into a disease classification, women can continue to be controlled politically, economically, and sexually. This opens the door for definitions of femininity and sexuality that are constructed by medical experts, rather than by women themselves. These are crucial insights, indicating how the feminist research aims to fully expose the medical construction of menopause. Yet, ironically, when it comes to the feminist research on menopause, the experiences of women themselves are generally left out of the endeavor.

Metaphors of Menopause in the Language of Feminist Literature

She stored up the anger
for twenty-five years,
then she put it on the table
like a casserole for dinner.

"I have stolen back
my life," she said.
"I have taken possession
of the rain and the sun
and the grasses," she said.

"You are talking
like a madwoman,"
he said.

"My hands are rocks,
my teeth are bullets,"
she said.

"You are my wife,"
he said.

"My throat is an eagle.
My breasts,
are two
white hurricanes," she said.

"Stop!" he said.
"Stop or I shall call
a doctor."

"My hair
is a hornet's nest,
my lips
are thin snakes
waiting for their victim."

He cooked his own dinners,
after that.

The doctors diagnosed it
common change-of-life.

(A portion of the poem "Midpoint" by Kathy Kozachenko, cited in Delaney et al. 237–38)

The metaphors found in the feminist studies of menopause are concerned with the need to offset the metaphor of menopause as breakdown
and disease promoted in the dominant scientific discourses. From the historical, cultural study of Delaney et al. metaphors have arisen, such as in
Kozachenko's poem (above) and Mary Winfrey's "At Menopause," in
which "the poet compares her body to a fruitless grapevine. Although the
grapes are gone, the vine continues to grow strong and to give shelter. . . .
the change of life can be an affirmation of our uniquely female experience
and an opportunity for new directions" (Delaney et al. 237, 239). This is a
portrayal similar to Zita's idea of a feminist tradition of menopause as
valorization.

Nurses, as health professionals, are challenged by MacPherson (1981)
to contribute to a growing body of literature that discusses menopause
positively and which may present the menopausal woman as a "hero." In
further writings, MacPherson (1985) has described how menopause
changed from a disease to a syndrome, which allowed for menopause to
become a treatable disorder. She has also described menopause as "a natural phase of the reproductive cycle and a part of the aging process" (17).

These feminist descriptions can be viewed as in opposition to the powerful images in the scientific or biomedical discourses about women and

menopause in our society. But in the realm of "power discourses" about menopause, their effects are weak compared to the effects of the dominant biomedical views of science, women, and menopause.

A Postmodern Paradigm

Postmodernism, a new world view, deals with the question of knowledge and social power in a postindustrial society (Lyotard). Scientific knowledge is viewed as a kind of discourse. However, scientific knowledge does not represent the totality of knowledge; it has always existed in addition to, in competition and conflict with, another kind of knowledge that Lyotard calls "narrative" knowledge. This knowledge includes notions of "knowing-how," "knowing how to live," "knowing how to speak," or auditory and visual sensibility, and so on (18).

Language assumes a new importance in postmodernism. Language is important, not because of its syntax and rules of grammar or the specifics of actual speaking, but insofar as it allows people to think, speak, and give meaning to the world around them. Discourse can be seen as a particular area of language use that may be identified by the institutions to which it relates, by the social position from which it comes, and by that position (such as scientist or expert) which it marks out for the speaker (Macdonell). Discourses, simply put, are language put into practice.

Basic to postmodernism is the tenet of context. The plurality of discourses and the impossibility of fixing meaning, once and for all, places any interpretation of language within the context of, at best, being specific to the discourses within which it is produced. Yet, language is the site of historically and socially specific discourses; this is where we perceive possibilities of social change through the range of discourses available to us. As Weedon suggests, it may be possible to transform the meaning of experience by bringing to bear a different set of assumptions on the language of the competing discourses.

Underlying Assumptions about Science. In postmodernism, assumptions about science flow from certain fundamental beliefs. First is the assumption that knowledge is fallible. It merely represents the best explanation available in which we trust enough to act. Second, knowledge is developed in a historical and cultural context. Historical knowledge helps to elucidate the unacknowledged conditions of research. Third, it is recognized that the values of the researcher have an impact on the choice of questions to study, as well as how to go about the study.

Fourth, the presumption is accepted that language is knowledge and that it is through the powerful discourses of a society that the subjectivity of an individual is formed in a way that is governed by specific social and historical factors. From the postmodern perspective, knowledge and power are viewed as opposite sides of the same coin; even the least of us is not powerless (Foucault 1977; Lyotard). Lastly, it is acknowledged that the scientific and medical literature is a reflection of the social and cultural conditions of a society and provides an insightful view of the larger society.

These assumptions allow for a study of language that encompasses both discursive and social fields, rather than that of individual men and women. Within this paradigm, "the rational individual is seen not as a proposition to be defended (or refuted), but as the consequence of social-historical processes, not as the intentional goal and underlying basis of history, but as its illusory result" (Poster 27).

Underlying Assumptions about Women. Differences between men and women are acknowledged in this paradigm. These differences are neither a means to explain nor a way to form behavior with a physiological base. Rather, the physiological differences are positive and mutually generative, not denied. "Different" does not mean unequal. "Difference" does not support theories in which men are the norm with women being the "other." A concern with difference can explore physiological differences, as well as those socially imposed upon women. The menstrual cycle is acknowledged and studied as women experience it and are concerned with it.

The historical and social discourses that are specific to women and menopause have helped to shape the experiences of women today. In this paradigm, women are assumed (a) to be equal to, but different from men; (b) to have experienced gender power imbalances in society as a result of unacknowledged conditions; and (c) to be capable of playing an active role in research addressing questions of concern to women (Dickson 1989).

Underlying Assumptions about Menopause. Menopause, in this paradigm, is assumed to be a physiological transition that all women will experience. It may occur naturally during midlife or be medically imposed at anytime in a woman's life. Women experiencing the menopausal transition are assumed to do so with a great deal of individual variation. What the experience is like is unknown, since normalcy of the transition has not been adequately addressed in research. The results of epidemiological studies tend to differ in regard to numbers and intensity of "symptoms" from those reported in the medical literature (Beyene; McKinlay et al.).

However, the assumption also is made that some women may have physiological changes that are problematic for them in maintaining their desired lifestyles.

A woman's response to this transition is a complex one, incorporating not only physiological dimensions, but social, historical, cultural, political, and economic dimensions as well. Therefore, any research designed to gain insight into the impact and scope of the menopausal transition should attend to physiological, social, historical, and cultural dimensions of knowledge and power. The postmodern paradigm provides the opportunity to develop a kind of research on menopause that (a) takes into account the historical and the sociocultural, as well as the biological, and (b) generates knowledge that represents *a* truth, not "*the* Truth," about menopause.

A Postmodern Study of Menopause. Exemplars of postmodern studies of menopause (and the only ones I am aware of) are in the work of Dickson (1989, 1990a, 1990b). In these studies, emerging from a postmodern paradigm, I explored the interrelation between the concept of knowledge in the scientific discourses and the concept of knowledge in the everyday discourses of midlife women regarding the closure of menstrual life. The data for analysis were twofold: the language of menopause in the scientific or biomedical literature of menopause, both present and past, and the language of a select group of midlife women.

Twenty interviews were conducted with eleven healthy, white, middle-class women, ranging in age from forty-seven to fifty-five years. The interrelation of the effects of professional "knowledge" upon midlife women was investigated through a discourse analysis comparing the scientific conceptualizations of menopause with the experiences described by the sample of midlife women. The outcomes of the research were identified as metaphors of menopause from the historical horizon and the everyday discourses, as well as those presented earlier from the biomedical, sociocultural, and feminist paradigms.

Metaphors of Menopause in the Language of Postmodern Research: The Historical Horizon. Several conceptualizations of menopause can be identified from the first published writings about menopause in the late 1800s. These conceptualizations lend themselves to particular metaphors that can be compared and contrasted to the differing metaphors from each time and from each paradigm. These metaphors represent, as have the others we have seen, the metaphors from the dominant discourses of that particular time in Western society.

The dominant conceptualization of menopause during the Victorian period was that of moral fault (Dickson 1989). The scientific view of womanhood that evolved was one in which the physician's would-be scientific views reflected and helped shape the social definition of the appropriate bounds of woman's role and identity. The scientific was called into play because women had become an issue, a social problem—something to be investigated, analyzed, and solved. Victorian society demanded that a woman be chaste, delicate, and loving. But, inside this discreet exterior and hidden deep within her lay her reproductive organs, which exercised a controlling influence on her whole body. Her reproductive organs were seen as "the source of her peculiarities, the center of her sympathies, and the seat of her disease. Everything that is peculiar to her springs from her sexual organization" (Smith-Rosenberg 1973, 59). Yet, with a life expectancy of forty-seven years, many woman did not live through menopause (Ehrenreich and English).

The first medical writings about menopause were by Tilt and appeared in France in 1851 (Wilbush 1980). By 1882 an edition had been translated into English for American audiences (Tilt). He used several metaphors as "it" was being given a name; they were "the end of the monthly" and "change of life" (Tilt). Other American doctors did not consider menopause a proper topic of discussion in medical circles. It was considered a normal process of aging by Mann, who wrote: "Take ten or twelve of the best known works on gynecology, and in most of them the word 'menopause' is not to be found in the index, and in none is it more than mentioned incidentally" (436).

However, as the century drew to a close, many physicians expressed the view that certain behavior (such as seeking too much education, attempts at birth control or abortion, seeking undue sexual gratification, insufficient attention to husband or children, or the advocacy of women's suffrage) caused a disease-ridden menopause (Smith-Rosenberg and Rosenberg). There was no doubt that childless women would suffer during menopause. They had thwarted the promise immanent in their bodies' design: they must expect to suffer (Dickson 1989). Several other metaphorical descriptions and names from the biomedical literature during this time were a "critical period of life" (Ricci); "climacteric" (Servinghaus), and "loss of power" (Smith-Rosenberg 1985).

As the twentieth century opened, the mantle of normalization passed from the family doctor to the specialist in diseases of the mind, the psychiatrist. Psychoanalytic "truth" was developed to support and reinforce the power of gynecology over women's lives. Attempts were made to convince women that many problems, including those attending menopause, were primarily intrapsychic, and "talking" could help to relieve those problems.

As the work of Freud was beginning to take hold in America, the closure of menstrual life became viewed as an event of loss and obsolescence (Dickson 1989). The scientific discourse of Helene Deutsch, a psychiatrist and student of Freud, was highly influential in setting new norms for the life of a menopausal woman. Deutsch presented a psychoanalytic interpretation of the psychology of women, illustrated with case studies from her psychiatric practice. The metaphors generated by her research were "natural end as servant of the species," "partial death," and "psychological distress."

The dominant conceptualization of menopause gleaned from the scientific discourses of this time can be expressed as "involutional melancholia." So prevalent was this "disorder occurring in the involutional period and characterized by worry, anxiety, agitation, and severe insomnia" (*Diagnostic and Statistical Manual of Mental Disorders* 36), that it became a psychiatric diagnosis. Now, in the official nomenclature of psychiatry, a direct relationship was formed between the menopausal transition or the involution of the uterus, and depression.

Women experiencing a difficult time at menopause were not those seeking education or birth control as earlier described, but those women with "immature personalities" (Petit). Other metaphors and descriptions that persisted from this period included "narcissistic mortification" and "inward anger and disappointment with one's self" (Klaus). These conceptualizations provided a different basis for the formulation and regulation of the "norms" of behavior for the menopausal woman, replacing the earlier "norms" set through the would-be science of the turn-of-the-century physicians, and set the stage for today's "hormone deficiency disease." However, it was the fundamental concept of womanhood as the persona of sexuality with an intrinsic pathology that allowed the conceptualization of menopause as disease to develop (Foucault 1980).

Metaphors of Menopause in the Language of Postmodern Research: The Everyday Discourse. As Foucault (1980) has carefully outlined, "each society has its regime of truth, its 'general politics' of truth: that is, the types of discourses which it accepts and makes function as true" (131). The scientific truth of today is that menopause is a "hormone deficiency disease." In the research I have conducted, evidence of the "truth effects" of the scientific can be heard in the voices of the women interviewed. But evidence of a resistance to this medicalization of menopause also can be heard in the voices. This can be considered an expression of the "woman in the body" (Martin).

Metaphors of menopause, representing both the truth effects and the woman in the body, can be identified from the language of the women interviewed. As women approach fifty and/or begin to notice some menstrual changes, there is a great deal of uncertainty that issues in wondering about and questioning of their experiences and their normalcy.

Some metaphors that the women used to describe this time in life include: "embarrassing and frustrating time," "hot flashes," "feeling blue" and "my change" (Dickson 1989). Others, reflecting a somewhat different perspective, include: "the beginning of a new life," "not a sick kind of thing," "terribly painless time," "end of childbearing years," "having energy," "enjoying life," "taking things into my own hands," and "feeling great" (Dickson 1989).

This postmodern analysis of the language of menopause lays the foundation for further research that would be freeing for women, that would help women gain a mastery of self through the knowledge of their experiences of menopause. The aim of this new research paradigm is to understand the experience of the "woman in the body," rather than seeing menopause through the lens of the biomedical paradigm.

Conclusion

The assumptions about science, women, the conceptualization of menopause, and the metaphors of menopause that are used to describe the results of the research from each of the four paradigms have been presented and discussed. The table summarizes, by paradigm, the assumptions and conceptualization or "reality" of menopause within each of the paradigms.

Comparing these differing views of the same experiences demonstrates how the specific assumptions about science link with the social ideology about women to provide (a) certain theoretical positions about menopause and (b) certain languages to describe menopause. For example, the presumptions about science in the biomedical paradigm are based on a linear, causal model, where facts are in relation to one another in combination with the social ideology of women as biological products of their hormones. These assumptions directly lead to the conceptualization of menopause as a hormone deficiency disease, which is reflected in the metaphors of the discourse.

In the sociocultural paradigm, the model of science is still a linear, causal one, but the variables of interest are social/cultural instead of biological. Women are defined in terms of responses to society and environ-

TABLE: Summary, by Paradigm, of the Assumptions about Science,
Women, and Menopause

Paradigm	Science	Women	The "Reality" of Menopause
Biomedical	Linear, causal: Facts in relation to one another; controlled variables; independent variable manipulation	Defined as: biological products of their hormones	Hormone deficiency disease. Symptoms can be reported
Sociocultural	Linear, causal: Persons in social interactions; field studies; attitudes and roles	Defined as: responses to society and environment	Natural process, socially constructed responses
Feminist	A critique that exposes social conditions that hinder communication and liberation; emancipatory	Defined as: equal worth in the market place of ideas; oppressed	Natural process of aging that encompasses social & class dimensions; rebirth
Postmodern	A textual analysis that attends to the social, cultural, and biological aspects; recognizes *a* truth; focuses on language in both social and discursive fields	Defined as: being shaped by historically & socially specific discourses	Plurality of experiences, no one truth, but evolving. Evidence of the "truth effects" and of "the woman in the body."

ment. Therefore, menopause is constructed as a natural process with problems related to socially constructed responses. Both of these paradigms of menopause research contain reductionistic approaches to research with the use of a linear, causal model. One, the biomedical paradigm, supports a biologic variable approach that reduces the study of women and "menstrual life to the study of ovary, uterus, or fluctuating hormones" (Voda and George 59). The other, the sociocultural, reduces the study of women to nonagents reacting to social and cultural, rather than biological, forces.

Research in a feminist paradigm attempts to support and describe women's experience during this time in life. It utilizes a sociocritique to expose the social conditions that hinder human communication and liberation. Women are defined as having equal worth in the marketplace of ideas, as well as having a history of oppression. Menopause is viewed as a natural process of aging that encompasses social and class dimensions. However, the incorporation of an essentialist perspective on gender and a discounting of the biological dimensions of menopause detracts from the usefulness of this research.

Finally, in the postmodern paradigm a different approach to knowledge and its generation is developed. The importance of language is emphasized in these postindustrial times when knowledge, rather than labor, is the mode of production. This allows for the methodology of a textual analysis that attends to the social, cultural, and biological dimensions of menopause. It acknowledges the plurality of discourses and multiple truths. Women and men are defined as being shaped by historically and socially specific discourses. Evidence in the metaphors of the historical horizon provide the basis for the evolving "truth." From the everyday discourse of women's voices, evidence can be found for the "truth effects" from the scientific discourses, as well as for the experiences of "the woman in the body."

Presenting the results of research in the form of its metaphors allows for a way of shedding new light on an existing phenomenon: menopause. From further studies, such as the one presented here, we can become increasingly conscious of our choices of research processes and the human nature of knowledge. This enables us to make decisions that ensure that our science (a) assumes the same reality as do our convictions, (b) accepts the same definition as our beliefs, (c) allows a similar understanding of the relationship between researchers and their objects of study, and (d) is directed toward ends similar to those of our practice (Moccia).

How we think about metaphors or meanings of a phenomenon determines how we use the words. For example, illness may be expressed as an enemy or as a comfort or as a weakness. The metaphors we hear shape how we perceive, interpret, or define symptom states (Lakoff and Johnson). Similarly, the metaphors of the discourses of menopause research contribute to the experiences of menopause for women. Defining menopause as a disease or as breakdown or as a developmental stage or as a social phenomenon or as rebirth will portend different experiences. It is possible, as Weedon suggests, that bringing to bear a different set of assumptions about science, women, and menopause in the discourses of menopause can transform the meaning of the midlife experiences for women. However, it is acknowledged that the "knowledge" of menopause discussed here represents a moment in history; the discourses and meaning of menopause are already changing.

REFERENCES

Allen, D., P. Benner, and N. L. Diekelmann. 1986. Three paradigms for nursing research: Methodological implications. In *Nursing research methodology: Issues and implementation,* ed. P. L. Chinn, 23–38. Rockville, Md.: Aspen.

Barrett-Connor, E. 1989. Long term estrogen replacement therapy: What we know and what we need to know. (Paper presented at the Eighth Conference of the Society for Menstrual Cycle Research, Salt Lake City, 1 June, 1989.)

Bell, S. E. 1987. Changing ideas: The medicalization of menopause. *Social Science and Medicine* 24:535–42.

Berg, G., and M. Hammar. 1985. Epidemiology of the climacterium. *Acta Obstetricia & Gynecologia of Scandanavica [Supplement]* 132:9–12.

Beyene, Y. 1986. Cultural significance and physiological manifestations of menopause: A biocultural analysis. *Culture, Medicine, and Psychiatry* 10:47–71.

Bleier, R. 1984. *Science and gender: A critique of biology and its theories on women.* New York: Pergamon.

Cohen, L. 1984. *Small expectations: Society's betrayal of older women.* Toronto: McClellan and Stewart.

Cook, T. D. 1983. Quasi-experimentation: Its ontology, epistemology, and methodology. In *Beyond method: Strategies for social research,* ed. G. Morgan, 74–94. Beverly Hills: Sage.

Delaney, J., M. J. Lupton, and E. Toth. 1988. *The curse: A cultural history of menstruation* (revised ed.). Chicago: University of Illinois.

Deutsch, H. 1945. *The psychology of women* (vol. 2). New York: Grune and Stratton.

Diagnostic and statistical manual of mental disorders (2nd ed.). 1968. American Psychiatric Association: Task Force on Nomenclature and Statistics.

Dickson, G. L. 1989. *The knowledge of menopause: An analysis of scientific and everyday discourses.* (Unpublished doctoral dissertation, University of Wisconsin-Madison.)

―――. 1990a. A feminist poststructuralist analysis of the knowledge of menopause. *Advances in Nursing Science* 12(3):15–31.

―――. 1990b. The metalanguage of menopause research. *IMAGE: Journal of Nursing Scholarship* 22(3):168–73.

Dosey, M. A., and M. F. Dosey. 1980. The climacteric woman. *Patient Counseling* 2(1):14–21.

Ehrenreich, B., and D. English. 1979. *For her own good: 150 years of the experts' advice to women.* New York: Doubleday.

Engel, N. S. 1984. On the vicissitudes of health appraisal. *Advances in Nursing Science* 7(1):12–23.

Fausto-Sterling, A. 1985. *Myths of gender: Biological theories about women and men.* New York: Basic Books.

Fee, E. 1986. Critiques of modern science: The relationship of feminism to other radical epistemologies. In *Feminist approaches to science,* ed. R. Bleier. New York: Pergamon.

Ferguson, K. J., C. Hoegh, and S. Johnson. 1989. Estrogen replacement therapy: A survey of women's knowledge and attitudes. *Archives of Internal Medicine* 149:133–36.

Flint, M. 1975. The menopause: Reward or punishment? *Psychosomatics* 16(4):161–63.

———. 1982. Male and female menopause: A cultural put-on. In *Changing perspectives on menopause,* ed. A. M. Voda, M. Dinnerstein, and S. R. O'Donnell, 363–75. Austin: University of Texas.

Foucault, M. 1977. In *Power/knowledge: Selected interviews and other writings 1972–1977,* ed./trans. C. Gordon. New York: Pantheon.

———. 1980. *The history of sexuality: Volume I: An introduction.* New York: Vintage.

Frey, K. A. 1981. Middle-aged women's experience and perceptions of menopause. *Women and Health* 6(1/2):25–36.

Genant, H. K., C. E. Cann, B. Ettinger, and G. S. Gordon. 1982. Quantitative computed tomography of vertebral spongiosa: A sensitive method for detecting early bone loss after oophorectomy. *Annals of Internal Medicine* 97:699–705.

Goldstein, M. Z. 1987. Aspects of gender and ethnic identity in menopause: Two Italian-American women. *Journal of the American Academy of Psychoanalysis* 15(3):383–94.

Harding, S. 1986. *The science question in feminism.* Ithaca: Cornell University.

Henig, R. M. 21 March 1988. Change of view on change of life. *The Milwaukee Journal,* 1D, 3D.

Hotchner, B. 1980. Menopause and sexuality: Gearing up or down? *Topics in Clinical Nursing* 1(4):45–51.

Iatrakis, G., N. Haronis, G. Sakellaropoulos, A. Kourkoubas, and M. Gallso. 1986. Psychosomatic symptoms of postmenopausal women with or without hormonal treatment. *Psychotherapy and Psychosomatics* 46(3):116–21.

Kaufert, P. A. 1982. Anthropology and the menopause: The development of a theoretical framework. *Maturitas* 4:181–93.

———. 1986. Menstrual changes and women in midlife. *Health Care for Women International* 7:63–76.

Kerlinger, F. N. 1986. *Foundations of behavioral research* (3rd ed.). New York: Holt, Rinehart & Winston.

Klaus, H. 1974. The menopause in gynecology: A focus for teaching the comprehensive care of women. *Journal of Medical Education* 49:1186–89.

Kuhn, T. S. 1970. *The structure of scientific revolutions* (2nd ed.). Chicago: University of Chicago.

Lakoff, G., and M. Johnson. 1980. *Metaphors we live by.* Chicago: University of Chicago.

Leininger, M. M. (ed.). 1985. *Qualitative research methods in nursing.* New York: Grune & Stratton.

Lennon, M. C. 1982. The psychological consequences of menopause: The importance of timing of a life stage event. *Journal of Health and Social Behavior* 23:353–66.

———. 1987. Is menopause depressing? An investigation of three perspectives. *Sex Roles* 17(1/2):1–16.

Lindsay, R., D. M. Hart, C. Forrest, and C. Baird. 1980. Prevention of spinal osteoporosis in oophorectomised women. *Lancet* 2:1151–53.

Lock, M. 1986. Ambiguities of aging: Japanese experience and perceptions of menopause. *Culture, Medicine, and Psychiatry* 10:23–46.

Lyotard, J. F. 1986. *The postmodern condition: A report on knowledge.* Minneapolis: University of Minnesota.

Macdonell, D. 1986. *Theories of discourse: An introduction.* Oxford: U.K.: Blackwell.

MacPherson, K. I. 1981. Menopause as disease: The social construction of a metaphor. *Advances in Nursing Science* 3(2):95–113.

————. 1985. Osteoporosis and menopause: A feminist analysis of the social construction of a syndrome. *Advances in Nursing Science* 7(4):11–22.

Mann, M. D. 1887. *A system of gynecology, by American authors.* Philadelphia: Lea Brothers.

Martin, E. 1987. *The woman in the body: A cultural analysis of reproduction.* Boston: Beacon.

McCrea, F. B. 1983. The politics of menopause: The "discovery" of a deficiency disease. *Social Problems* 31(1):111–23.

McKinlay, J. B., S. M. McKinlay, and D. J. Brambilla. 1987. Health status and utilization behavior associated with menopause. *American Journal of Epidemiology* 125:110–21.

McKinlay, S. M., and J. B. McKinlay. 1973. Selected studies of the menopause. *Journal of Biosocial Science* 5:533–55.

Moccia, P. 1988. A critique of compromise: Beyond the methods debate. *Advances in Nursing Science* 10(4):1–9.

Morgan, G. 1983. Research strategies: Modes of engagement. In *Beyond method: Strategies for social research,* ed. G. Morgan, 19–42. Beverly Hills: Sage.

Nachtigall, L. E. 1987. Estrogen replacement: Which postmenopausal women benefit? *The Female Patient* 12(8):72ff.

Nicholson, L. J. 1990. Introduction. In *Feminism/Postmodernism,* ed. L. J. Nicholson, 1–16. New York: Routledge.

Petit, M. D. 1955. Management of the menopause. *The Medical Clinics of North America* 39:1725–31.

Polit, D. F., and S. A. LaRocco. 1980. Social and psychological correlates of menopausal symptoms. *Psychosomatic Medicine* 42(3):335–45.

Popkewitz, T. S. 1984. *Paradigm and ideology in educational research: The social functions of the intellectual.* London: Falmer.

Posner, J. 1979. It's all in your head: Feminist and medical models of menopause (strange bedfellows). *Sex Roles* 5:179–90.

Poster, M. 1984. *Foucault, Marxism and history.* Cambridge, U.K.: Polity.

Ravnikar, V. A. 1983. When your patient faces menopause. *Patient Care* 17(11):91–103.

Ricci, J. V. 1945. *One hundred years of gynaecology: 1800 to 1900.* Philadelphia: Blakiston.

Riggs, B. L., and J. Melton. 1986. Involutional osteoporosis. *The New England Journal of Medicine* 314:1676–84.

Riggs, B. L., H. W. Wahner, L. J. Melton, III, L. S. Richelson, H. L. Judd, and K. P. Offord. 1986. Bone loss in the axial and appendicular skeletons of women: evidence of substantial vertebral bone loss prior to menopause. *Journal of Clinical Investigations* 77:1487–91.

Russett, E. 1989. *Sexual science: The Victorian construction of womanhood.* Cambridge: Harvard University.

Servinghaus, R. L. 1948. *The management of the climacteric: Male or female.* Springfield, Ill.: Charles C. Thomas.

58   Cultural Constructions, Policy, and Practice

Smith-Rosenberg, C. 1973. Puberty to menopause: The cycle of femininity in nineteenth-century America. *Feminist Studies* 1(3/4):58–73.

———. 1985. *Disorderly conduct: Visions of gender in Victorian America.* New York: Oxford.

Smith-Rosenberg, C., and C. Rosenberg, 1984. The female animal: Medical and biological views of woman and her role in nineteenth-century America. In *Women and health in America,* ed. J. W. Leavitt, 12–27. Madison: University of Wisconsin.

Tilt, E. J. 1882. *The change of life in health and disease* (4th ed.). New York: Bermingham.

Uphold, C. R., and E. J. Susman. 1981. Self-reported climacteric symptoms as a function of the relationships between marital adjustment and childrearing stage. *Nursing Research* 30:84–88.

———. 1985. Child-rearing, marital, recreational and work role integration and climacteric symptoms in midlife women. *Research in Nursing and Health* 8:73–81.

Voda, A. M., and T. George. 1986. Menopause. In *Annual Review of Nursing Research* (vol. 4), ed. H. H. Werley and J. J. Fitzpatrick, 55–75. New York: Springer.

Walfisch, S., H. Antonovsky, and B. Maoz. 1984. Relationship between biological changes and symptoms and health behaviour during the climacteric. *Maturitas* 6:9–17.

Weedon, C. 1987. *Feminist practice and poststructuralist theory.* Oxford, U.K.: Blackwell.

Weideger, P. 1976. *Menstruation and Menopause.* New York: Alfred A. Knopf.

Whatley, M. H. 1986. Integrating sexuality issues into the nursing curriculum. *Journal of Sex Education and Therapy* 12(2):23–26.

Wilbush, J. 1980. Tilt, E. J. and the change of life (1857)—the only work on the subject in the English language. *Maturitas* 2:259–67.

———. 1982. Historical perspectives: Climacteric expression and social context. *Maturitas* 4:195–205.

Wilson, H. S. 1989. *Research in nursing* (2nd ed.). Menlo Park, Calif.: Addison-Wesley.

Wilson, R. A., and T. Wilson. 1963. The fate of nontreated post-menopausal women: A plea for the maintenance of adequate estrogen from puberty to the grave. *Journal of the American Geriatric Society* 11:347–62.

Zita, J. N. 1993. Heresy in the female body: The rhetorics of menopause. In *Menopause: A midlife passage,* ed. J. C. Callahan, 59–78. Bloomington: Indiana University Press.

Heresy in the Female Body: The Rhetorics of Menopause

Jacquelyn N. Zita

One woman I talked to said her doctor gave her two choices for treatment of her menopause: she could take estrogen and get cancer or she could not take it and have her bones dissolve.

—Emily Martin

Sickness is rarely a plain event.

—Susan Sontag

A new female body inhabits the West. This woman escapes estrus, lives longer, bleeds more, breeds less (if at all), refuses domestic asylum, and with age increasingly may become poor, expendable, and readily forgotten. She is a woman likely to live for more than a quarter of a century after menopause. Compared to a premodern foremother, whose reproductive life of five offspring in a hunting and gathering society was likely to involve four years of pregnancy, fifteen years of lactational amenorrhea, and four years of menstruation, a modern woman, who frequently carries two pregnancies to term with little or no breast-feeding, menstruates for about thirty-five years or approximately half a lifetime, nine times as long as her early foremother (Lander 170). These changes in menstrual bleeding and postmenopausal longevity are recent evolutionary developments in the human female.

A modern demographic profile of postmenopausal women in the United States reveals another socioevolutionary change—postmenopausal women exist in increasing numbers and with decreasing social value. Whereas in 1900 there were more elderly men than women, in 1982 there were sixty-seven men to every one hundred women over the age of sixty-five, and forty-three men to every one hundred women over the age of eighty-five. The population of women older than forty-five has grown dramatically, with more than 22 million women between the ages of forty-five and sixty-four and 12.8 million women older than age sixty-five. These women make up over three-fourths of the older-than-sixty-five population living below the poverty line, with a poverty rate for this age group of women double that for men (MacPherson 1985, 13). The economic oppression of postmenopausal women is further enhanced by an ideology of sexist ageism that views the older female body as a surface for the metaphors of disease, disability, and medical dependency, calling into question, with increasing age, female entitlement to state-sanctioned public power. An older woman in our culture runs a high risk of being a poor woman and of being perceived as a menopausally damaged woman. This culturally constructed and painful reality is not only metaphysically odd but politically crafted.

In thinking about menopause as a site for competing rhetorics of interpretation, I think of the body as a text where these rhetorics contend for privileged readings. These readings often culminate in evaluations or diagnoses, as in "this body is sick," "this body is dysfunctional," "this body is deviant," "this body is normal, healthy, natural," and so on. One reads the body as a text with its presentation of signs, symptoms, incidental alterations, and this seems a simple matter of opening the book of flesh and finding what is there. With this approach, the body's connections to larger cultural processes—to social relations, symbol cultural systems, codes of disciplines that affect the body, and institutionalized conventions of gender and sexuality—are obscured by a privatized relation of text to reader or body to expert. Here is where I find political concern. Monolithically negative rhetorical readings of the menopausal body, I will argue, are designed to obscure a larger cultural picture—namely, the material relations between the sexes—by reading the body as a text that unfolds its own negative meanings. These meanings, I will argue, are at least in part a creation of a masculinist gerontocracy invested in the penultimate disempowerment of the female sex.

I will explore this idea from several different angles. First, I will examine how menopause has been interpreted by three different rhetorical strategies: biological essentialism, scientific reductionism, and feminist valorization. I use the term "rhetoric" to sidestep questions on the adequacy of scientific theorizing on menopause, questions which have been carefully examined by others (Voda and George; Goodman 1980, 1982; Woods; Koeske; McKinlay and McKinlay 1973; Dickson 1990, 1993)*, because I

---

*After completing this essay, I had an opportunity to read Geri Dickson's "Metaphors of Menopause: The Metalanguage of Menopause Research," also included in this anthology. I was pleased to find that our approaches to the bio-cultural aspects of menopause are very similar. However, my insistence on a feminist approach, which I do not see as ontologically

am particularly interested in how language is used to negotiate and interpret women's subjective menopausal experience and how this is related to the "body politic" of a male gerontocracy. Second, I will examine three different concepts of "the body" presupposed by these rhetorical strategies. These differences are important, since reference made to "the body" seems to assume a shared or commonly understood thing in the world. My analysis will show that this assumption is misleading and that shifting concepts of "the body" create theoretical and political incompatibilities between these rhetorical strategies, with the appeal to women's authority on menopausal experience constituting an important oppositional discourse for "remaking" the meanings of menopausal bodies and for understanding the body as a discursively constituted thing. I conclude with several challenges to traditional views on menopause designed to sabotage the discursivities that produce the aged female body. These include (1) the elimination of demeaning gender bias in the rhetorics of menopause, (2) the improvement of life circumstances for postmenopausal women, and (3) the termination of a metaphysical misogyny hostile toward the changing physical integrity of the female flesh and inimical to the dignity, power, and knowledge won by the aged crone. These strategies focus on the materialities of language and socioeconomic conditions as a way of changing the bodies of lived experience and improving the quality of female life.

The Rhetorics of Menopause

The body is a site where different meanings compete for reference. This does not deny that the term "menopause" refers to a bodily event—"the final cessation of menstruation"—but it suggests that the meanings of that event, its cultural, historical, and personal interpretations, are dependent on the rhetorical strategies used to re/present and interpret all of what it is. I will examine three such competing rhetorics and their definitions of menopause: menopause as the loss of true femininity (bio-gender essentialism), menopause as a dysfunctional or functionless state (scientific reductionism), and menopause as a "natural" life transition (feminist valorization).

---

essentialist as Dickson does, marks our difference. I concur with Diana Fuss, who argued that it is possible to use essentialist language for pragmatic and political ends or for strategic and interventionary values without becoming reactionary or metaphysically overloaded. Unlike Dickson, I shy away from the postmodernism of Lyotard because of a need to stay close to a materialist analysis of the social relations between the sexes. For my in-progress critiques of postmodernism, see Zita (1988 and 1992).

Biological Gender Essentialism

While the term "essence" refers to what makes a thing what it is (its "essential qualities"), "biological essentialism" refers to what a thing essentially is in biological terms. "Woman," accordingly, both *is* her biology and is determined by her biology. Wilson, in his book *Feminine Forever*, considers a woman's Pap smear a count that "answers one of the most crucial questions that ever confront a woman. It tells her whether her body is still feminine, or whether it is gradually turning neuter" (91). Menopause is perceived as an estrogen-deficiency disease, a deviation from the norms of true femininity, restorable through estrogen replacement therapy. According to Wilson, "estrogen therapy doesn't change a woman . . . it keeps her from changing" (53). Failure to make this intervention results in lost gender identity: "no woman can be sure of escaping the horror of this living decay . . . even the most valiant woman can no longer hide the fact that she is, in effect, no longer a woman" (43). From this perspective, the body is a biological text, "woman" *is* her biology, and menopause is a deviance from the gendered norm of true femininity, a loss of womanhood produced by a biological change.

The estrogen-restored woman is importantly a "sexually restored woman" (21), and like her estrogen-rich former self, she is "capable of being physically and emotionally fulfilled by her husband or lover and least likely to go afield in search of casual encounters" (65). For Wilson, a heterosexual and monogamous femininity, that "subtle and almost metaphysical factor—woman's total femininity" (26) serves as the norm against which menopause is contrasted. This is amplified by his use of oppositional metaphors, such as life and death, youth and decay, wet and dry, sexed and neutered. The loss of vigor, youth, fluidity, fertility (equivalents of "womanhood") portends the coming of death, decay, dryness, and neutered asexuality, a movement from the norm of feminine heterofecundity to the horror of menopausal senescence. The gendered body appears as a biologically bound entity, which at menopause commits a heresy against its own nature. Wilson encourages steroid restoration, arguing that "women have a right to remain women. They should not have to live as sexual neuters for half their lives" (25).

From the perspective of Wilson's bio-gender essentialism,
(1) A woman's body is a biological text.
(2) The essence of "woman" (her biological reproductivity and true femininity) is determined by her biology.

(3) Menopause converts a woman into a "neuter" or a nonwoman.

(4) Menopause is a deviance in gender ontology requiring medical intervention.

Scientific Reductionism

Scientific reductionism differs from bio-gender essentialism in isolating the body as an organic entity with its own internal biological laws of well-functioning. Instead of "normalizing" the body with respect to gender, the body is "normalized" with respect to the medical norm of "health" (Judd; Vermeulen; Nachtigall). Rather than being described as "neutered," the menopausal woman is said to suffer a "loss in health status." Medical description depicts menopause in terms of "dysfunction," "syndromes, symptoms, and disease," or acute events such as a "crisis" or "catastrophe"—categories of deviation measured against the norm of health rather than true femininity. The causes of dysfunction are found *in the body,* usually following a reductivist explanation which isolates causal factors on the micro-levels of bodily substance. In the case of menopause, cause for deviation from the norms of well-functioning is located in hormonal changes. The logic of such explanation is often simplistically reductive, since hormonal changes associated with menopause are also associated and correlated causally by hypothesis with the presentation of negative "symptoms" in a menopausal body. Clinical writing often uses adjectives such as "hypogonadal," "castrate," or "estrogen-deficient" (Voda and George) to refer to a postmenopausal woman, suggesting once again that she is not quite a complete woman. However, most scientific reductionist readings of the body are more "clinically objective": the definition of menopause as a "disease" (MacPherson 1983) or "dysfunction" or a dysfunctional "functionlessness" (Martin) signifies menopause as a problem requiring medical intervention.

From the perspective of scientific reductionism,

(1) A woman's body is a biological text.

(2) The status of that body is measured with respect to the norms of internal well-functioning or "health."

(3) Menopause is seen as a deviation from the norms of well-functioning caused by an internal disturbance or malfunctioning.

(4) Menopause is a dysfunction in the body's health status requiring medical intervention.

Both biological essentialism and scientific reductionism locate meno-pause as a situation *in the body,* caused by internal dysfunction. Most frequently the therapy of preference used by these practitioners is hor-mone replacement therapy, a treatment which decreases the number of presenting symptoms and "evidences the symptoms" (in a circular fashion, those which appear to be hormone-dependent). From both of these per-spectives, authority to decipher the body's meanings and status is granted to a medical practitioner, who "looks at" and examines the female subject, often equating her speaking and behaviors with symptoms or signs of bod-ily dysfunction. In both biological essentialism and scientific reductionism, the structural authority of the body justifies the validity of the interroga-tion. In other words, the body's ideological function is to exist in nature, siphoned off from cultural, historical, and social contexts, and to provide a prediscursive object for clinical inquiry. Since menopause is construed as a biological event, it seems to be a universal sex-linked and body-bound natural phenomenon. Thus, menopause as a hormone-deficiency malady is referred back to the biology of the female body, implicating that body, and in particular female gonads, as the source of this disturbance.

From a physical point of view, these two rhetorics can be used to jus-tify an exceedingly negative portrait of the late endocrine effects of meno-pause in the female body (Utian 1282):

Late Endocrine-Related Climacteric Symptoms

Target Organs	Possible Symptom or Problem
Vulva	Atrophy
	Dystrophy
	Pruritis vulvae
Vagina	Dyspareunia
	Blood-stained discharge
	Vaginitis
Bladder and urethra	Cystourethritis
	Ectropion
	Frequency and/or urgency
Uterus and pelvic floor	Uterovaginal prolapse
Skin and mucous membranes	Atrophy, dryness, or pruritis
	Easily traumatized
	Loss of resilience and pliability
	Dry hair or loss of hair
	Minor hirsutism of face
	Dry mouth

Target Organs	Possible Symptom or Problem
Vocal cords	Voice changes—reduction in upper register
Cardiovascular system	Atherosclerosis, angina, and coronary heart disease
Skeleton	Osteoporosis with related fractures Backache
Breasts	Reduced size Softer consistency Drooping
Neuroendocrine	Hot flushes, psychological changes

Feminist Valorization

> *I feel that I am expanding in my*
> *life more than I ever have before.*
> *My wisdom, my experience make*
> *my judging of situations much*
> *richer than when I was younger.*
> *. . . the best is yet to come sexually.*
>
> —*Rosetta Reitz*

Menopause has existed in human females as long as there have been menstruating women who cease to ovulate. Menopause as a difficult or easy life transition has also been part of these life cycles. What has not always existed is the historical invention of menopause as a "corridor of disease, dysfunction, and devaluation" and the construction of "the menopausal body," through a compendium of case studies, replete with etiologies, patient histories, tried remedies, and an array of "symptoms and signs" which refer back to a state of dysfunction in the body. Any female body which enters "the menopausal corridor" becomes a body saturated with the meanings of menopause which unfold in temporal successions of bodily and psychological changes that are recodified as "symptoms." Medical inquiry persistently refers back to an event—the menopause—as a way of understanding the textual meanings of the changing female body.

Feminist critique of the rhetorics of menopause has challenged this cultural construction of menopause by calling into question those experts who claim exclusive privilege in reading, "remedying," and fixing "the menopausal body" and by challenging certain metaphysical assumptions underlying the construction of such a body. Raising the question of who has a right to interpret the meanings and status of the body, feminist approaches to menopause expand the location of authority, often "giving voice" to and valorizing female experiences of menopause. The "monolithic menopausal body" as a master text for reading the meanings of many female experiences of "the menopause" is replaced by a variety of bodies, experiences, and voices which escape diagnostic closure and even celebrate menopause as a positive life transition. These voices have either been silenced or erased by a medical gaze that sets its sights on the horrifying dangers of the menopausal corridor.

Feminist deconstruction of this rests upon empirical research which reveals that women do not necessarily see menopause as a distressing event (Frey; Neugarten et al.; McKinlay and Jefferys; Goodman 1982). Karen Frey found that forty to sixty year old women currently going through menopause show no greater frequency of physical symptoms than pre- or postmenopausal women (34). Her data also suggest that experiences of menopausal distress may be related to class identity, with women in professional occupations having the highest wellness orientation, the secretarial-clerical group second, homemakers third, and blue-collar workers fourth (Frey 33). As Judyth Reichenberg-Ullman has pointed out, "contrary to the medical community's belief that menopause—categorized as a 'deficiency disease'—has a negative impact on women's lives, a study found that among women experiencing natural menopause (as opposed to surgically induced) only 3% were regretful, 17% had mixed feelings, 41% were neutral, and 39% were relieved" (Reichenberg-Ullman 80).

The fetishized focus on menopause as dis-easing or dis-abling has relied almost exclusively on the voices of women in clinical populations—women who have come to doctors seeking relief for bodily complaints (McKinlay, McKinlay, and Brambilla). Rather than colonizing these complaints as evidence of universal female defect, feminists have challenged the quick-footed reductionist moves which seek explanation in the body's interior. An alternative reading of the body points to areas outside of skin and flesh for an understanding of female somatic experience. The body under the sign of "menopause" may signify for many women distressing life transitions which implode the meaning of menopause. Events such as children's leaving home; changes in domestic, social, and personal relationships; changes in identity and body image; possible divorce or widowhood; new experiences of retirement; and increasing anxiety about aging, dying, and losing friends, loved ones, and financial security can coincide with the time of menopause in a woman's life. For women this perhaps troubling time of life can profoundly diminish a sense of well-being and self-worth and lend a negative interpretation to the experience of menopause (Bart). It is a time of life redoubled in negative meanings with ageist metaphors applied to the female body (Cohen; MacDonald; Copper)—a woman becomes "castrated," asexual, unfeminine, a dried-up bag of bones, a dislocated body in her passage through the menopausal corridor. While it is true that some women, but not all, and not the majority, it seems, experience menopause as a dreadful, painful, and frightening event, a new alternative reading of these "symptoms" connects them to a larger picture, to a culturally constructed life-precipice that terrorizes women with the loss of prestige, status, visibility, and value during the last quarter-century of female life.

Cross-cultural studies tend to confirm that the meaning of menopause depends on dimensions of cultural practice and sense-making which inform the lived particularity of menopause as well as its generic representations within a given culture. Several studies show that in cultures where postmenopausal women gain status, menopause is not associated with disease or dysfunction (Beyene; Flint; Walfish et al.; Goodman et al; Davis). For example, in Beyene's studies of the Mayan Indians, physicians, midwives, and women in general all agreed that " . . . menopause in the Mayan culture is unrecognized except as marking the end of menstruation and childbearing" (Beyene 58), and that Mayan "women welcomed menopause and associated this stage with being young and free" (60). Alternatively, negative menopausal experience can receive positive evaluation, as seen in the complicated case of the Newfoundland fishing village, studied by Davis, where menopause is viewed as a series of cultural gains and losses, a suffering required to bring women into higher social status, " . . . for one gets high status from stoically enduring life's lot" (83). In a culture such as ours, where menopause portends possible loss in social status, dominant representations of menopause are those of disease or dysfunction, with any associated pain and distress labeled menopausal symptoms.

Feminists have countered our culture's negative view of menopause by reconstruing menopause as "a transitional phase," "a developmental stage" or "a positive or at least a neutral experience." In *Menopause: A Positive Approach,* Rosetta Reitz compares her birth experience with menopause: "Why am I looked on with value when my body is going through one *natural* function, then, twenty years later, looked on as valueless when my body is going through *another natural function?*" (17, emphasis mine). The semantic shift to adjectives such as "natural," "neutral," and "positive" challenges negative definitions of "menopause" and expands the scope of the term "woman." As Reitz comments, "I accept that I'm a *healthy woman* whose body is changing" (181, emphasis mine). In this rhetorical strategy, the female body is seen as going into a new stage of life, where "your ovaries do not fail at menopause; they merely go through their *natural process*" (15, emphasis mine). Ontological priority is given to the body's full life cycle, allowing that postmenopausal and old women are still "women," not "sexual neuters," "gonadal casualties," or "weirdly shrunken men."

Use of the word "natural" does not necessarily refer to a new essentialism (Fuss). Having a negative experience of menopause does not mean, however ironically, that a woman has done something "unnatural." Use of the word "natural" is meant to contest the meanings of "woman" that identify womanhood with reproductively fertile years and relegate postmenopausal women to the abhorrently unnatural "other," to be hidden from sight or fixed by steroids, surgeries, and addictive disciplining of female flesh. To deem "menopause" a natural life transition is to make space for older females in the registers of womanhood. To consider menopause a "natural" event in the lives of women also opens up a listening space for the voices of many women who missed the "clinicalized" experience of menopause. Diversity, multiplicity, possibility, and power emerge against the background of a medically monolithic and essentialized menopausal body. When these new voices escape diagnostic closure, they support oppositional and alternative readings of the body and the sense we make of our embodied experience. Menopause becomes a personal, physical, cultural, and political event, located both inside and outside the physical boundaries of the body and inside a larger body politic.

From the perspective of feminist valorization,
(1) The body is a bio-cultural text; in part biologically given and in part culturally constructed in its meanings.
(2) This body is "naturalized" by its relationship to a woman's entire life cycle and is construed as the site for contesting struggles over the meanings and readings of menopause.
(3) Menopause is a "natural life transition" which is variously experienced by women; some may experience this transition as difficult and disabling and others may find it a positive and easy experience.
(4) Interventions to help women adjust to the bodily changes that occur in the menopausal years are multiple; they may include symbolic, personal, spiritual, and political interventions, as well as a variety of physical remedies.

In summary, a feminist approach challenges the authority of other rhetorics by letting women speak from their own experience and by valorizing what women say, not just those women from selected clinical populations. In such research, there is less symptom reporting, a more commonly shared positive experience of menopause, and an understanding that female menopausal complaints are at least partially dependent on sociocultural, historical, and personal life transition factors. The body is seen as a medium between nature and culture, and female experience of menopause is seen as influenced, though not exclusively, by the cultural meanings given to gender, sexuality, female-specific aging, and other social differences. In contrast to the norms of youthful femininity (bio-gender essentialism) and hormonal high-functioning (scientific reductionism), a feminist approach advocates integration, multiplicity, and resistance: self-acceptance of body image and life cycle process, defiance against social practices which disempower older women, and celebration of the transforming landscapes of the female flesh.

"The Body" of Menopause

> *Perhaps we need a moratorium on saying "the body."*
>
> *When I write "the body," I see nothing in particular. To write "my body" plunges me into lived experience, particularity.*
>
> *To say "the body" lifts me away from what has given me a primary perspective. To say "my body" reduces the temptation to grandiose assertions.*
>
> —*Adrienne Rich*

To use the term "the body" is to use a generic word, applicable to anything that is human or living or for that matter, merely occupying space. "The body," used generically, is not necessarily gendered, sexed, racialized, or even particularized, although differences among and between bodies are used to make such distinctions. "The body" homogenizes these differences, allowing for generalization over many individual bodies, while recognizing that individual narrative accounts of "my body" may be unique and contextually dependent on my cultural and historical location, as well as the kind of body I live in. References to "the body" in the three rhetorics of menopause I have examined refer to different sorts of generalized bodies, revealing, I believe, different political agendas that motivate these rhetorics.

"The body" of bio-gender essentialism contains "genderedness" within it, an internal essence regulated by hormones. These biochemical controls determine not only primary and secondary physical sex characteristics of the body, but also the behaviors, attitudes, and desires expected of women. From this perspective, "the body" controls both its phenotypic and behavioral display of sex difference. Menopause or the decline of estradiol in the female body is seen as contrary to nature, a heresy in the female body. From a political point of view, the body's rescue is carried out by medical experts, who fix the body and repair its deficiencies, leaving women dependent on these remedies and invested in a frantically perceived "inferiorization" which comes with age. Because these attempted restorations of youth and beauty ultimately fail, it is women in the end who fail, and fall.

"The body" in scientific reductionism is perceived as a self-contained living organic entity, governed by its own laws of internal well-functioning and equilibrium. Sex differences between bodies are cast as differences in bodily parts, substances (genes, tissues, hormones, organs), or their distribution. "Well-functioning" and "normal" are terms applied to the body to show how body parts and substances function together (and to what end) and how to "read the body" for symptoms or signs of internal malfunctioning. This reading of the body is generally reductionist, starting from the presentation of symptoms, lab test results, instrumental readings, and focuses inward toward the molecular or cellular levels for explanation. "The body" of scientific reductionism is literally bound by its skin and by a concept of its self-contained organicity. From this perspective, menopause marks a change in the body's internal functioning, a change in hormonal profiles, from which proliferate a number of symptoms and dysfunctions, requiring medical intervention. Knowing the body requires special knowledge of the body's internal functioning, a knowledge not readily available in our everyday lived experience of the body. From a political point of view, this medicalization of the body carries many of the same dangers as that of bio-gender essentialism, albeit, hidden in the cloak of objectivity and rationality.

"The body" in feminist valorization plays a number of roles. Like "the body" of biological essentialism, it provides a place where gender happens, but new theorizing suggests that gender may be seen as enacted or performed through the body not because of the body (Butler). Like "the body" of scientific reductionism, it is a place where structure and function in the flesh are maintained by internal mechanism, but not the place where every condition that we come to know as "the menopause" is constituted.

When many women, especially women responding in nonclinical situations, give their own personal accounts of menopausal experience, the totalizing diagnosis of "menopause as disease" and the much-advertised dangers of "the menopausal corridor" are challenged by conflicting accounts drawn from women's personal experiences. These accounts, if taken seriously, create the possibility for new forms of authority and new meanings for menopause. From a political point of view, this rhetorical strategy leads to the self-empowerment and collective empowerment of women, and like other aspects of the women's health movement, it spurs the development of grass-root and home-bound techniques for coping with difficult menopausal experience (Clay; Reitz; Greenwood; Doress and Siegal; Whitlock) and the development of a new language for the telling of menopause (Skultans; Wilbush).

From a feminist approach, "the body" is seen as less self-contained, less defined by its skin boundaries, and less able ontologically to encapsulate the meaning of gender. "The body" is seen as a location, situated between nature and culture, as a thing both biologically given and culturally constructed, having both structure and function and providing a surface upon which cultural texts are written, contested, and rewritten. Menopause, accordingly, is a biological event occurring inside the body and coinciding with various meanings and interpretations originating outside the body. Feminist valorization creates a wider semantic and political space for interpreting this body. This does not necessarily foreclose all possibilities of reductionist diagnosis, but it asks the diagnostician to listen in different ways and become more culturally reflexive. Thus, the appearance of "symptoms," "complaints," and "dysfunctions" may possibly, though not necessarily, indicate internal malfunction. Such signs may also indicate the need to ask further questions about the way in which a woman is reading her own body, the rhetorical strategies she has available for making sense of what is happening in her body, and her internalized attitudes toward menopause and postmenopausal women.

Menopause is a physical event in the body, but its interpretation as *the loss of true femininity,* as *disease, dysfunction, or functionlessness* or as *a natural life cycle transition* with complicated political consequences determines how it is experienced and perceived. It is not the case that these three rhetorics rely on the same concept of the body in referring to "the body." Further, this is not to deny that some women experience severe hot flashes, painful vulvar dryness, or mood adjustments to hormonal remodeling of the body, but severity in these conditions is not the rule, and living through these changes can be described with differing rhetorical strategies which call upon different means for effective survival. What feminist valorization reveals is a discursively constituted body, which is as much a product of its biology as it is a product of institutional forces and cultural meanings imposed upon and disciplined into the flesh of our experience. In the monolithically essentialized body of some medical thinking, "the menopause" becomes a theoretical term creating a web of intelligibility and diagnosis for changes occurring in "the menopausal body." In such thinking, a multiplicity of bodily changes are derived from a singularly distilled category—"the menopause"—which fastens meaning and suspicion onto ever-increasing and multiply diverse phenomena. The valorization of many women's voices, speaking from the category of menopause, contests this negative semantic space and the historical construction of "the monolithic menopausal body." In this sense, the strategies of feminist valorization bring into focus the phenomenon of my body, plunged into "lived experience, particularity" (Rich 215).

Obviously, the rhetorical strategy of valorization can be called "feminist" because it lends itself to the self-empowerment and collective empowerment of women, while challenging unhealthy and unreflective forms of female dependency on medical authority and misogynist readings of menopausal experience. This approach is also feminist in its cultural critique of the discursively constituted menopausal body as a product of social, sexual, and material relations between the sexes. This is a body produced by a particular body politic.

Changing the Body Politic

> While symptoms of illness are
> "undeniably biological phenomena
> experienced by individual bodies,
> they are also something else besides;
> they are coded metaphors capable
> of speaking eloquently to troubling
> aspects of social life by covertly
> expressing feelings, sentiments, and
> ideas that are normally disallowed."
>
> —Nancy Scheper-Hughes

In my analysis of menopause so far I have suggested that different ways of rhetoricizing menopause result in different concepts of "the body" and that by giving women agency and voice to rewrite the scripts and meanings imposed upon the female body, a new sense of menopause can emerge, one that can inspire celebration and revitalization of this life-cycle transition. There is yet another way of "reading the body" from a feminist perspective. The symptoms of illness can be read, as Scheper-Hughes suggests, as metaphors for troubling social conditions, not easily brought to conscious awareness. The body could be seen as "speaking to us" about its social and personal situation, rather than blankly reflecting its interior density. The symptoms point to a problem in the body politic, requiring a social rather than an exclusively medical diagnosis. The term "body politic" refers to a discursive cultural practice in which bodies are controlled and regulated, so that individuals and populations maintain and continuously produce the social, political, economic, and sexual relations of production and reproduction. From what we know about sexism, heterosexism, racism, classism, ageism, ableism and other socially significant oppressions, these relations of production and reproduction are asymmetrical and defined by an unequal distribution of power. What is produced and reproduced in such a body politic is social power and bodies infused with it or its lack; the aggregates of all these bodies crystallize into the macro-level relations of race, gender, class, and other significant social divisions of domination and subordination.

Modern male gerontocracy is a body politic defined by the different meanings given to age in the two sexes: males have more opportunity to acquire social power and capital with the coming of age while females are "culturally and socially enfeebled" with the coming of age. In modern male heteroeconomies of the body, the youthful female body represents sex, causes its arousal, and is responsible for the provocation and constraint of male sex drive. The aged female body blocks such arousal and meaning patterns, since the ideology of ageism represents the old female as asexual if not antisexual. The sensuous confirmation needs of heteromasculinity read the aged female as a negative sign. She is gladly left out of the picture, except for benign grandmotherly roles, gladly forgotten, and gladly replaced by younger females, whose bodies match the Platonized ideal of unchanging and "unaging" female beauty, captivating the psychic needs of a culturally constructed heteromasculinity (Stoltenberg). The crone becomes spectoral, an appearance without substance, the open secret of female aging. The agedness of masculinity becomes the masthead of political power.

Although these changes in gender status are cultural events, orchestrated by social institutions and ideologies which also favor class, race, and other distinctions, they often work at odds with the purported biological durability and longevity of female bodies. Why, we might ask, has so much attention been given to the negative effects of menopause and much less medical and cultural concern given to its positive values? Why has so little attention been given to the changes associated with male climacteric and its attendant, often life-threatening, prostate complications? Why isn't female longevity amplified by cultural rhetorics awarding this somatic durability with political channels of power and higher social status? Age affects both sexes, but why are the more odious meanings of ageism unevenly dumped on the female body? The construction of "the monolithic menopausal body" is a political deployment, not by accident first historically "implanted" on the bodies of upper-class European women (Smith-Rosenberg; Dickson, this anthology). It is designed to disempower the aged female (Kaufert and Gilbert; MacPherson 1981, 1985; McCrea). The idea of blaming the female body for its own loss of social power is useful to a male gerontocracy, where aged virility for males of privileged social status amasses greater social and capital power. The loss of reproductive capacity in women is interpreted as the loss of social capacity; literally in some cases it is a loss in socioeconomic identity, a fall from fertility and "estrogenated" soma to the aged crone, whose spectral aura of poverty, dryness, depletion, and "ugliness" are fetishized as reflections of death and disappearance.

On the other hand, the postmenopausal woman poses a serious threat to the authority and autonomy of a body politic which has always justified women's dependency and secondary social status as a function of female reproductivity, the quintessential cultural meaning of "womanhood." The change in female flesh marked by menopause and its embodied metaphors causes disturbance in an androcentric culture, uneasy reminders of the unharnessed female flesh and of old women, potentially powerful, autonomous, and wise. Yet the postmenopausal body is overdetermined by imagery signifying shame and disempowerment. These images make it easier to live in a male body, drawing on the social graces of age to seduce more youthful female bodies into possession, while pushing *old woman* to the wayside. It is her refusal that must be silenced as a "symptom."

Concluding Matters

I would like to end this essay with a few suggestions for social change, suggestions for altering "the body" by changing the body politic of our male gerontocracy. Again, this is not to say that the meanings we read into menopause are completely determined by social scripts and relations of power. "The body" is an organic entity with structures and functions which can break down and go awry; but it is also an object which acquires social meaning and social location through cultural practices, which in turn can profoundly affect the body's health, well-being, and our lived interpretation of our bodies. In accordance with feminist valorization, the remedies for this ailing gerontocracy are multilayered and laced with strategies for female empowerment. These strategies intervene at various material levels that discursively constitute the meaning and status of our gendered and aging bodies.

(1) *Matters of Language and Representation.* We must make every effort to eliminate the demeaning gender bias which appears in the rhetorics of menopause: from the rhetorical bias which refers to the postmenopausal woman as "castrate," "estrogen-deficient," or "functionless," to the research bias which overemphasizes the negative aspects of menopause and postmenopausal existence. We must promote and fund positive menopausal research and construct positive rituals and representations for this life transition.

(2) *Matters of Power.* We must fight to improve the social, political, and personal life circumstances of postmenopausal women, since the culturally constructed "enfeeblement of the female sex" is largely a political and economic strategy which enforces the rule of a male gerontocracy. Perhaps we have something to learn from the social, political, and economic mechanisms used to empower the aged male and how race and class affect its simple functioning. My suggestion is not that we create a new female gerontocracy, but we must challenge the mechanisms of injustice that currently exist and bring all aged crones into view, not as spectral shadows, but as women in our full presence, substance, and power.

(3) *Matters of Metaphysics.* Finally, we must challenge the metaphysical misogyny which defines "woman" by her reproductive capacity, a *misogyny* which is everywhere present in women's obsessive concern with "the youthful perfect body" and a *metaphysic of essence* which underlies the monolithic construction of the menopausal body and the inescapable odium of the menopausal corridor. Womanhood does not stop at menopause. It is empowering to assert that a postmenopausal woman does not cease to be a woman. As Cindy Patton has suggested in her recent work on the HIV body, "attention and surveillance, silence and relinquishing of control over one's own meanings are discursive effects symptomatic of relations of power" (3).

To change the meanings and norms of "woman," to include the rambling and unfettered spaces of the female flesh, to allow for female lifelong dignity and power, and to honor the increasing wisdom of older women with political access—and all of this regardless of race or class—would significantly alter the landscapes of our body politic. This requires radical changes in the meanings of menopause and a complete deconstruction of "the monolithic menopausal body" and the negativity of "the menopausal corridor." To deconstruct the meanings of menopause in a male gerontocracy is to construct a social and cultural space for the empowerment of crones. The matter of words in this political project is indeed part of all the matter needed for this rearrangement of flesh and meaning. My hope is that more powerful and unruly women will emerge from this conceiving—old, wise, and furiously heretical.

REFERENCES

Bart, P. B. 1972. "Depression in Middle Aged Women." *Women in Sexist Society.* Ed. V. Gornick and B. K. Moran. New York: New American Library. 163–86.
Beyene, Yewoubdar. 1986. "Cultural Significance and Physiological Manifestations of Menopause: A Biocultural Analysis." *Culture, Medicine, and Psychiatry* 10:46–71.
Butler, Judith. 1990. *Gender Trouble: Feminism and the Subversion of Identity.* New York: Routledge.
Clay, Vidal. 1977. *Women: Menopause and Middle Age.* Pittsburgh: KNOW.
Cohen, L. 1984. *Small Expectations: Society's Betrayal of Older Women.* Toronto: McClellan and Stewart.
Copper, Baba. 1988. *Over the Hill.* New York: Crossing.
Davis, Dona Lee. 1986. "The Meaning of Menopause in a Newfoundland Fishing Village." *Culture, Medicine, and Psychiatry* 10:73–94.
Dickson, Geri. 1990. "The Metalanguage of Menopause Research." *IMAGE: Journal of Nursing Scholarship* 22.3:168–73.
———. 1993. "Metaphors of Menopause: The Metalanguage of Menopause Research." In *Menopause: A Midlife Passage,* ed. J. C. Callahan, 36–58. Bloomington: Indiana University Press.
Doress, P., and D. Siegal. 1987. *Ourselves Growing Older.* New York: Simon and Schuster.
Flint, M. 1974. "Menarche and Menopause in Rajput Women." *Dissertation Abstracts International* 34, 12B.
———. 1975. "The Menopause: Reward or Punishment?" *Psychosomatics* 16:161–63.
Frey, Karin. 1981. "Middle-Aged Women's Experience and Perceptions of Menopause." *Women and Health* 6.1/2:25–36.
Fuss, Diana. 1989. "The 'Risk' of Essence." *Essentially Speaking.* New York: Routledge. 1–21.
Goodman, M. J. 1980. "Toward a Biology of Menopause." *Signs: Journal of Women in Culture and Society* 5:739–53.

————. 1982. "A Critique of Menopause Research." *Changing Perspectives on Menopause.* Ed. A. M. Voda, M. Dinnerstein, and S. R. O'Donnell, 273–88. Austin: University of Texas Press.

Goodman, M. J., C. J. Stewart, and F. Gilbert. 1977. "Patterns of Menopause: A Study of Certain Medical and Physiological Variables among Caucasian and Japanese Women Living in Hawaii." *Journal of Gerontology* 32.3: 291–98.

Greenwood, S. 1984. *Menopause Naturally: A Preparation for the Second Half of Life.* San Francisco: Volcano.

Judd, H. L. 1976. "Hormonal Dynamics Associated with the Menopause." *Clinical Obstetrics and Gynecology* 19:775–88.

Kaufert, Patricia A., and Penny Gilbert. 1986. "Women, Menopause and Medicalization." *Culture, Medicine, and Psychiatry* 15E:7–21.

Koeske, R. K. 1982. "Toward a Biosocial Paradigm for Menopause Research: Lessons and Contributions from the Behavioral Sciences." *Changing Perspectives on Menopause.* Ed. A. M. Voda, M. Dinnerstein, and S. R. O'Donnell, 3–23. Austin: University of Texas Press.

Lander, Louise. 1988. *Images of Bleeding: Menstruation as Ideology.* New York: Orlando.

MacDonald, Barbara. 1983. *Look Me in the Eye: Old Women, Aging, and Ageism.* San Francisco: Spinsters.

MacPherson, K. I. 1981. "Menopause as Disease: The Social Construction of a Metaphor." *Advances in Nursing Science* 3.2:95–113.

————. 1983. "Feminist Research Methods: A Nursing Paradigm Shift." *Advances in Nursing Science* 5.2:17–25.

————. 1985. "Osteoporosis and Menopause: The Social Construction of a Syndrome." *Advances in Nursing Science* 9.4:11–22.

Martin, Emily. 1987. "Medical Metaphors of Women's Bodies: Menstruation and Menopause." *The Woman in the Body: A Cultural Analysis of Reproduction.* Boston: Beacon. 27–53.

McCrea, Frances B. 1983. "The Politics of Menopause: The 'Discovery' of a Deficiency Disease." *Social Problems* 31.1:111–23.

McKinlay, S. M., and M. Jefferys. 1974. "The Menopausal Syndrome." *British Journal of Preventive Social Medicine* 28.2:108–15.

McKinlay, J. B., S. M. McKinlay, and D. J. Brambilla. 1987. "Health Status and Utilization Behavior Associated with Menopause." *American Journal of Epidemiology* 125.1:110–21.

McKinlay, S. M., and J. B. McKinlay. 1973. "Selected Studies of the Menopause." *Journal of Biosocial Sciences* 5:533–55.

Nachtigall, L. E. 1987. "Estrogen Replacement: Which Postmenopausal Women Benefit?" *The Female Patient* 12.8:72ff.

National Women's Health Network. 1989. *Taking Hormones and Women's Health: Choices, Risks, and Benefits.* Washington, D.C.: National Women's Health Network.

Neugarten, B. L., V. Wood, R. J. Kraines, and B. Loomis. 1963. "Women's Attitudes toward the Menopause." *Vita Humana* 6.3:140–51.

Patton, Cindy. 1990. *Inventing AIDS.* New York: Routledge.

Posner, J. 1979. "It's All in Your Head: Feminist and Medical Models of Menopause (Strange Bedfellows)." *Sex Roles* 5:179–90.

Reichenberg-Ullman, Judyth. 1992. "Menopause Naturally." *Natural Health* 22.2:75–80.

Reitz, R. 1977. *Menopause: A Positive Approach.* New York: Penguin.

Rich, Adrienne. 1986. "Notes toward a Politic of Location." *Blood, Bread, and Poetry: Selected Prose 1979–1985.* New York: W. W. Norton. 210–31.

Scheper-Hughes, Nancy. 1988. "The Madness of Hunger: Sickness, Delirium, and Human Need." *Culture, Medicine, and Psychiatry* 12:429–58.

Seaman, B., and G. Seaman. 1977. *Women and the Crisis in Sex Hormones.* New York: Bantam.

Skultans, Vieda. 1970. "The Symbolic Significance of Menstruation and the Menopause." *Man* 5.4:639–51.

Smith-Rosenberg, Carroll. 1974. "Puberty to Menopause: The Cycle of Femininity in Nineteenth-Century America." *Clio's Consciousness Raised.* Ed. Mary Hartman and Lois W. Banner. New York: Harper and Row. 23–47.

Sontag, Susan. 1988. *Illness as Metaphor.* New York: Farrar, Strauss, and Giroux.

Stoltenberg, John. 1990. *Refusing to Be a Man: Essays on Sex and Justice.* New York: Meridian.

Utian, W. H. 1987. "Overview of Menopause." *American Journal of Obstetrics and Gynecology* 156.5:1280–83.

Vermeulen, A. 1976. "The Hormonal Activity of the Postmenopausal Ovary." *Journal of Clinical Endocrinology and Metabolism* 42:247–53.

Voda, A. M., and T. George. 1986. "Menopause." *Annual Review of Nursing Research.* Vol. 4. Ed. H. H. Weerley and J. J. Fitzpatrick. New York: Springer. 55–75.

Walfish, S., A. Antonovsky, and B. Maoz. 1984. "Relationship between Biological Changes and Symptoms and Health Behavior during the Climacteric." *Maturitas* 6:6–17.

Weideger, Paula. 1975. *Menstruation and Menopause: The Physiology and Psychology, the Myth and Reality.* New York: Delta.

Whitlock, Evelyn. 1988. *The Calcium Plus Workbook.* New Canaan, Conn.: Keats.

Wilbush, Joel. 1981. "What's in a Name? Some Linguistic Aspects of the Climacteric." *Maturitas* 3:1–9.

Wilson, R. 1966. *Feminine Forever.* New York: M. Evans.

Wilson, R., and T. Wilson. 1963. "The Fate of Non-Treated Postmenopausal Women." *Journal of American Geriatric Society* 11:347–62.

Woods, N. F. 1982. "Menopausal Distress: A Model for Epidemiologic Investigation." *Changing Perspectives on Menopause.* Ed. A. M. Voda, M. Dinnerstein, and S. R. O'Donnell. Austin: University of Texas Press. 220–47.

Zita, Jacquelyn. 1988. "The Feminist Question of *The Science Question of Feminism.*" *Hypatia: Special Issue on Feminism and Science* 3.1:157–68.

———. 1992. "The Male Lesbian and the Postmodernist Body." *Hypatia: Special Issue on Feminism and Science* 7.4:106–27.

Who Needs a Menopause Policy?

Jill Rips

Can we invent other practices that treat difference as just the variety of human experience, rather than the basis for dividing people into the class of the normal and the class of the abnormal?

—Martha Minow

The ways in which menopause or menopausal women are conceptualized help to determine the organization of policy and services targeted at women of menopausal age. My question is: What does a feminist perspective on menopause imply socially, economically, and politically in terms of the empowerment of women?

In preparing this paper, I anticipated producing a neat and tidy feminist policy on menopause. Believing that much of the denigration of midlife women, and women more generally for that matter, results from pejorative stereotypes generated by a white, male-dominated power structure, I thought the direct antidote would be to bring menopause "out of the closet." Such a policy would illuminate menopause for what I thought it was, a rite of passage to a new life stage with its attendant functions and exigencies. It would be a policy that made no excuses for hot flashes in public or for a sexuality not tied to reproduction; no apologies for aging and the special needs of midlife women, nor for their loss of reproductive capabilities. My first stumbling block, however, was the question of why there currently was no nexus of medical, social, and welfare policies dealing with menopause. Was the lack of policy the result of neglect or conscious choice? Was it due, perhaps, to an unwillingness to make distinctions, based upon fear of some possibly deleterious consequences of labeling midlife as something special?[1] Thus the intent to formulate policy led to a more fundamental questioning of not only the utility of such an effort, but also of the negative side-effects potentially engendered by a policy that would establish a special category justifying, even implicitly, considering midlife women as something apart, that is, different. As a consequence, this paper raises more basic questions than it answers, but I hope it will be the beginning of a constructive discussion regarding a feminist policy on menopause.

With regard to policy, I will not focus on the question of routine treatment for menopause or, more specifically, hormone replacement therapy. Neither will I discuss establishing a policy regarding the issue of informed consent; that is, of a woman making an informed decision about treatment based on knowledge of the latest studies, her individual physical status and value system, and notions of personal and collective risk. These issues are addressed elsewhere in this volume.[2]

Instead, I will address how the organization of knowledge with its concomitant categories of meaning is as much based on ideology as on what might be described as "pure" reason. Ideology shapes, supports, and reflects social relations and infrastructure. A particular structuring of reality (for example, one in which women are subordinate to men) is responsible for a still all too prevalent ideology of female inferiority based on notions of pathology, weakness, or irrationality. Rather than looking for the presence or absence of a reified phenomenon, whose delineation may in itself be problematic, we should instead proceed more cautiously and empirically and see which life events emerge as salient or as crises for individual women. For, by even accepting the labels "menopause" or "midlife," we may be accepting the biomedical conceptualization of women's lives, if not the current content of that conceptualization. I will explore how the definitions and descriptions created for menopausal or midlife women are the result of larger issues of gender and social relations. Do we need to foster more positive images of menopausal women so as to contribute to improvements in their status and power, or should we aim directly for women's empowerment, trusting that more positive views of midlife women will come in its wake?

I shall alternate throughout this paper between the terms "menopausal" and "midlife" women. This is partly due to finding neither term aptly descriptive and partly to my general ambivalence about labeling. "Menopause" is meaningful when discussing, for example, vasomotor changes. On the other hand, much of what gets thrown into the cauldron popularly called "menopausal syndrome" I believe to be the result of ideology rather than physiology.

Some might argue that "midlife" should be to "menopause" as "gender" is to "sex," with the former in each case denoting social roles and the latter referring to biological or physiological characteristics. One problem with this approach is that although midlife occurs in both men and

women, its more distended, less "eventful" physical manifestations in men
have not been tied, either popularly or by medical providers, to psychological, developmental, or social manifestations of behavior. At least with
puberty, there is more even-handed insistence upon the salience of raging
hormones in both sexes—albeit that in boys hormones are said to produce
predictable "boys-will-be-boys" behavior, while in girls they are said to
cause behavior which is simultaneously more "demure" and "seductive."
Yet the cross-cultural literature suggests that puberty is associated with an
extremely broad range of behaviors. There are cultures in which "adolescence" as a problem is not a part of the social construction of puberty:
one merely passes into biological adulthood. This should inspire us to
imagine what it might be like to separate the biological changes of menopause from their presumed psychosocial concomitants. If, for the sake of
convenience, we use the term "midlife" to connote a segment of the life
cycle as process, it is worth bearing in mind that, for many women, this
segment does *not* mark a major disjuncture from what precedes or follows.
The term can be useful if we consciously keep its meaning broad enough
to encompass the vast range of women's actual experiences. Thus, it serves
as a shorthand for the chronology of women's lives from their middle to
late forties through their fifties. What we must guard against is attaching
additional connotations to the term or allowing them to adhere. For if by
"midlife" we mean to denote a particular psychological phase or demarca-
tion of uniformly experienced social roles (as postulated in much life stage
theory), then the term will be less useful for *explaining* women's roles and
experiences and will instead *constrain* our understanding of them.

Before going further, let me digress to remark on my personal interest
in menopause. As in most peregrinations that take on importance in our
lives, my initial introduction to menopause emerged from the personal.
My characteristically healthy, energetic mother became depressed and en-
ervated during her menopause, which commenced during my sophomore
year in college. Living half a country away, I could do little more than offer
support and, as a budding anthropologist, take mental notes and wonder if
it had to be so. Dealing only with the personal at that moment, I reserved
my questions about what occurs at the interstices of biology and culture
for later.

Having tucked them away, my questions about menopause reemerged
in graduate school where the personal became the political as cross-
cultural and historical variation challenged the hegemony of a western
biomedical model of menopausal experience. The ethnographic record in
all of its variety offered a plethora of cultural constructions of a biological

process. It soon became clear to me that menopause, like other physiological life events such as birth, death, and menarche, takes on different meanings in different cultural contexts, as well as multiple meanings within a single society. So my once personal quest to understand my mother's menopausal experience was expanded, using menopause as a lens through which to question broader topics of gender roles, ageism, and the medical-industrial complex.

Growing interest in menopause can be found in several sectors in our society. In particular, interest has been raised by the graying of the founders of the women's health movement and by the pharmaceutical industry, which recognizes an essentially limitless market in promotion of hormone replacement therapy from premenopause through postmenopause. However the topic should be of concern to all who are interested, theoretically, in how value attaches to an attribute and, practically, in what roles those values play in determining the social relations between the definers and those defined by the attribute. Through the study of menopause as a social construct, we can question the dichotomies that have importance in our society. The topic highlights the oppositions between female and male, old and young, reproductive and postreproductive, abnormal or pathological and healthy.

I wish to be clear that I believe for some women the physiologic changes associated with menopause, such as the hot flush or flash, as well as the personal and social meanings attached to those changes, can be extremely debilitating. But this is not the case with all women; and a primarily negative experience with menopause should not be assumed to be universal, as several other papers in this book make clear. Variety and multiplicity of experience should be tenable without requiring the incorporation of those experiences as inseparable or natural aspects of the definition.

What Does Marking of the Categories "Menopause" and "Midlife" Imply?

We name to distinguish. Minow suggests that labeling and naming differences to distinguish favors boundaries rather than relationships. Naming isolates not only those labeled as "different," "marginal," or "other," but also those who do the naming. It establishes a false sense that it is the "marginal" person who is dependent upon the namer, when actually there is a mutual interdependency. "Man" opposes and yet is dependent upon "woman," as is "adult" with "child," "white" with "black," and "boss" with "worker." Such oppositions often point to power imbalances or hierarchies in our society.

Demarcations or categorizations can be used as a means of self-assertion or as a means to keep others from sharing or gaining access to sources of power. Typically, the initial source of such categorizations is *not* those named, but those who wish to distinguish themselves and, thereby, retain sole access to power through the exclusion of others denoted by the distinction made. Minow points out that even in cases where members of minority groups or groups of less power have attempted to rename themselves, they may share in or have incorporated the power structure, if not the exact terms, of the larger society of which they are also members. "For this very reason, the efforts to rename oneself may be circumscribed by the attitudes and authority of those who have defined the difference" (Minow 5–6).

"Woman" names a distinct category, and emphasizing distinctness can be a means of self-revelation and celebration for women.[3] It also allows women to make the best of an unequal situation, since often this insuperable separateness is merely a manifestation of gender prejudice on the part of men. But overemphasis of differences in midlife, or at any life stage, may be more likely to engender distrust than to empower women. A perspective based on shared human attributes may be more likely to foster equality and mutually recognized interdependence between men and women at midlife. Let us consider some possible ramifications of taking menopause or midlife as a special category and whether this difference or special status serves to empower women in the long run.

Because so little has been written with regard to policy for menopause, we will have to proceed by analogy, relying on historical examples. Three examples come to mind in which struggles have occurred over creation of special policies for women: (1) protective labor laws for children and women, (2) pregnancy as "disability" in the work place, and (3) premenstrual syndrome, or PMS, and menstruation. The "correct" feminist position on the first two examples is not obvious. I will discuss PMS, which has been more thoroughly researched than menopause, later when considering the applicability of cultural constructions of menstruation for menopause.

The question is whether specialized legislation or policy helps women or works against them. To protect women and children by precluding them from harmful work conditions seems, on the surface, benign and laudable. However, such policies have served to foster a two-tiered pay scale that often reserves higher-paying work for men. In workplaces that might prove harmful to a woman's reproductive system, women are sometimes given the "choice" of sterilization or no job, even when it is known that men working in the same environments are also put at reproductive risk by an environmental hazard.[4] A genuinely equitable policy would require work conditions that are safe for both women and men rather than allowing women's exclusion. A workplace policy that treats pregnancy as disability is equally problematic. On one hand it recognizes that some pregnant women have special needs and limitations, which seems positive. However, to view pregnancy as disability supports the categorization of women as weaker and inferior to men and pregnancy as pathology, rather than as a natural process.

Menstruation: A Case in Point

Menstruation, another biological phenomenon that is enmeshed in symbolic meaning, is contiguous to menopause in terms of biological chronology. The recent collection, *Blood Magic: The Anthropology of Menstruation*, demonstrates that menstruation is accorded negative or positive value, or is viewed neutrally (i.e., taken as merely biological occurrence) in different cultural contexts (Buckley and Gottlieb). For example, Laura Appell shows that the Rungus of Borneo ignore menstruation, other than as an instance of elimination of body fluids. Menstrual blood is not seen as polluting in this culture, where other body byproducts and emissions of human blood are believed to be dangerous or dirty. Appell attributes this anomalous lack of menstrual symbolism partly to shared power between men and women, which is reflected by the Rungus' social organization. Rungus' gender roles are equally valued, even though not the same. Similarly, these roles are interdependent, with each requiring the cooperation of the other, and there is no separation of public and private spheres.

In contrast, in *Images of Bleeding: Menstruation as Ideology*, Louise Lander documents the transformations of menstrual ideology within American and British culture from religious moralizing, to proscriptive behavior, to psychologizing and, ultimately, to biologizing, with the biomedical marketing of menstruation as disease with PMS. Lander notes that menstruation is not an anomaly, but is just another example within chronobiology of the innumerable human rhythms that are based on either daily, monthly, or yearly cycles. "Cyclicity is an integral part of the fabric of earthly existence, not an aberrant characteristic of the second sex" (146). Thus the question becomes: Why are women's hormonal rhythms singularly treated as anomalous despite contrary scientific evidence? The medical position might suggest that women have been or should be limited in opportunity because of biology, whereas Lander suggests that women are subordinated for other reasons and biology is called upon as justification for inequity.

Finally, the push to include so-called premenstrual syndrome (PMS), under the title of Late Luteal Phase Dysphoric Disorder (LLPDD), as the only diagnosis peculiar to women to appear in the appendix of the recent edition of psychiatry's *Diagnostic and Statistical Manual* (DSM III-R) may foreshadow a similar designation for menopause. The creation of a diagnosis based on the experience of a few allows for the potential limitations of *all* women by questioning *all* women's psychological stability. The ovarian determinism of the nineteenth century seems to have been replaced by hormonal determinism in the late twentieth century.

Although not to the same extreme, a similar scenario is occurring with regard to depression held to be specific to menopause. Although included in DSM-I and II, so-called Involutional Melancholia was eliminated from DSM-III, mainly as a result of the general defeat of the psychoanalytical school within psychiatry and the ascendancy of diagnoses related to observable criteria (Lerman). However, the urge within mainstream psychiatry to find biochemical explanations for all behaviors, along with the emphasis on hormonal explanation within medicine in general, has left the door open for the reintroduction of menopausal depression. This association of depression with menopause is viewed as the outcome of shifts in hormone levels, rather than as the effect of women's accession of lower self-worth resulting from society's view and treatment of menopausal and aging women. The question of etiology between feelings and hormones is crucial here. Medicine has typically taken hormones to be the cause of changing emotions. But why should it not be the case that emotions contribute to hormonal changes? Certainly the well-documented, but poorly understood phenomena, stress-delayed cycle and menstrual synchrony, raise questions regarding the direction of causality between psychological and physiological phenomena.[5]

How do the preceding considerations inform the issue of policy on menopause? With LLPDD and Involutional Depression we see the potential for attributing to hormones or psyches the depression or rage that may well be engendered by socially limited roles. The byproducts of gender inequality come to be regarded as individual difficulties. Consequently, individual solutions are sought for collective problems resulting in individual acquiescence and acceptance, rather than group empowerment.

Lander's piece asks why female rhythms are of special interest to and subject to manipulation by the medical community, when chronobiology in men does not equally capture their attention. Finally, Appell's discovery that menstruation as an unmarked category among the Rungus is the result of gender symmetry and mutual male/female interdependence suggests that the latter causes the former. Where there is gender equality, the facts of female biology are not burdened with extraneous meanings, rather than the reverse. A special emphasis on female biological distinctiveness is associated with an exacerbation, rather than a mitigation, of gender inequality. The implications are profound for empowering women and promoting gender symmetry in our own society.

The Consideration of Policies and Their Categorizations

Having considered some of the ramifications of policies specifically targeted at women in areas other than menopause, let us now see what different menopausal policies might mean for midlife women, given certain commonly accepted dichotomies.

Reproductive vs. Postreproductive: A policy based on the reproductive/postreproductive dichotomy would call for special health-care services, such as menopause clinics. By accepting a medical categorization of women on the basis of their menstrual status, we may end up defining women in terms of their reproductive status—a definition that surely does not serve women well, either in their reproductive or postreproductive years.[6]

Is there a need for specialized care for menopause? Despite the medical and popular view that menopausal women suffer considerably from both somatic and psychological symptoms, the epidemiological evidence from prospective, population-based samples indicates that menopause for most women produces neither poorer health status nor increased utilization of health care services (Lennon; McKinlay et al. 1987a,b). Despite the fact that most women do experience some vasomotor menopausal symptoms, these are generally limited and not perceived by them as requiring medical or psychological intervention. Thus, it seems that calling for specialized menopause clinics is neither necessary nor desirable.

Old vs. Young: Another way to define menopause is in terms of its place in life's chronology. Thus menopause as a species of "old" is pitted against "young." I was interested to discover that the overwhelming regret stated by women in a menopause self-help group I attended was that of being seen as old. To identify themselves as menopausal meant that they could no longer mask their age. Despite how young and energetic they may have looked or felt, to publicly acknowledge their menopausal status was to define themselves in society's eyes as old. Men as a collective, they pointed out, had no comparable benchmark that marked them as old.

The question arises of whether there is anything peculiar about menopause that establishes it as a rite of passage from young to old. Or are aging changes more gradual and extremely variable? Those concerned with methodological issues in menopause research have been careful to point out the necessity of designing studies to distinguish the effects of aging from those of menopause (e.g., Goodman). Even designating those nonphysiological changes of menopause as part of midlife can be very problematic. Critiques of life stage theory suggest that those characteristics and experiences attributable to midlife are based on limited white, middle-class experience. In discussing the social construction of age, Lichtman states, "there are of course changes which occur in the body over time, but it is very difficult to say what these are independent of cultural symbolization; and even if it were possible, the meaning of the natural is always given by our society" (72).

Thus, to create special policy for menopausal women as a marked category in opposition to young women is to ascribe needs or particular attributes where they may or may not be experienced. To be sure, for some women midlife may be a fundamentally different life stage, with children leaving home and more time to focus on personal growth and needs. And some women may use midlife as a rite of passage, as the only available means to act on desired changes in their lives. However, for those women whose childcare duties do not end in the middle years or whose grown children are financially unable to leave home, midlife may involve no major break in daily life. Women who never had children will similarly see no major changes in that arena of social roles. If the purpose of menopausal policy is to improve women's empowerment during their middle years, those changes will not come about through a limited struggle which pits their lot against that of younger women, but through a collective effort that refutes both sexism and ageism.

Male vs. Female or Normal vs. Abnormal: Finally, another way to structure the menopause policy debate is to pit female against male. A focus on the differences rather than on the similarities between males and females in terms of health care needs tends to reaffirm the biomedical model, which takes the male as normal and that which does not conform (the female) as abnormal or "sick." I have already mentioned that both men's and women's bodily processes are dictated by cyclicity or biorhythms. Similarly, the behaviors of men, like those of women, are just as much a product of their emotions as of their endocrine systems. Although the immediacy of challenges from the right have forced feminists to focus on those areas where a woman's health needs are different from those of a man (e.g., the right to control her own body through the right to legal abortion), a woman's health needs extend beyond care of her reproductive system.

All of this is not to suggest that there are no differences between the health care needs of men and women. Certain protocols for treatment may be helpful within a context of nonspecialized clinics. A woman should be offered treatment options, informed of the known and potential benefits and risks of each, and allowed to be an active decision-maker and participant in her own treatment. However, this right to truly informed consent should be afforded to all within the health-care system, men and women alike.

The needs of menopausal women who are without a private caregiver may be different from those of their middle- and upper-class counterparts. Medically indigent women in midlife do not benefit from those medical and social services afforded to women in their reproductive years (through contraceptive or prenatal services) and older women (through Medicare). The only care many women receive is tied to pregnancy and/or contraception. Once they no longer need such care, all medical service may cease until some medical crisis occurs. While not old enough to qualify for Medicare, it is extremely difficult for a midlife woman to qualify for Medicaid if she is not blind, disabled, or with children under 18.

Clearly there is a need to validate personal experience and to demystify the physiological process of menopause in all its variety. The New York City Department of Health's Pregnancy Testing Centers reported that women in their middle years often presented themselves for pregnancy testing, unaware that their amenorrhea was the result of menopause. In most cases, these women were essentially uninformed about menopause, its manifestations and expected course. Hence the development and dissemination of multilingual, easily legible, nonjudgmental, and informative health-education literature on menopause should be a priority for the women's health movement.

However, many of the health-care needs of midlife women that are not currently met result not from biological differences but from lack of resources, caused by pay inequity with midlife men or by no or inadequate health care insurance. Eighty-five percent of private health insurance in this country is group coverage provided by employment, and since women are more likely to be employed in low-paying, part-time, and nonunionized jobs, they are less likely than men to have health benefits (Older Women's League). Besides employment, insurance coverage for midlife women is often a function of their marital status; that is, married women are more likely to be covered than widowed or divorced women, regardless of their employment status. Midlife women earn one-third the income of midlife men and are more likely to be uninsured than their male counterparts (Older Women's League). Still, to me, the answer for the medically indigent or underinsured is equal pay for equal work and a national health service or insurance, which would benefit everyone, not just women.

Conclusion

Thus the end of my search for a feminist policy on menopause turns out to be its beginning, like the ouro boros, or alchemical dragon, that is nourished through consuming its own tail. We have come full circle from speculating about the need for a separate menopause policy to a call for more generic policies. While not denying difference, we need not seek special status for menopausal women. What we need are not only more positive definitions of menopause; with social equality negative stereotypes will give way. As I come full circle, it seems to me that the creation of alliances based on shared concerns of race, class, and sexual freedom will do more than a menopause policy to empower women and to free both men and women from the shackles of sexism and ageism which are so integral to the biomedical definition of menopause.[7]

NOTES

1. I have the work of Martha Minow, discovered during my final edit, to thank for theoretically grounding my hunches. Minow refers to "the dilemma of difference," which has the potential to recreate stigma "both by ignoring and by focusing on it" (20). "The dilemma of difference grows from the ways this society assigns individuals to categories and, on that basis, determines whom to include in and whom to exclude from political, social, and economic activities. Because the activities are designed, in turn, with only the included participants in mind, the excluded seem not to fit because of something in their own nature" (21).

2. See Part II.

3. Some critics of deconstructionism reject a reductive notion of "woman" which purports to understand women's experience. Such singular notions of "woman" dismiss the variety of women's experience based on other attributes, such as race or class, which may subsume or confound gender in particular contexts (Minow).

4. This issue was recently decided by the Supreme Court in *International Union et al. v. Johnson Controls,* which struck down Johnson Controls' exclusionary policy. The Court itself notes that men are put at reproductive risk by the same environmental toxin (lead) used in the argument for excluding women. Exclusion from particular occupations on the basis of genetics or physiology is not limited to women. The Dupont Corporation has excluded African Americans with Sickle Cell Trait from employment. While the exclusion was purported to be in the interest of the health of potential employees, the policy effectively served to bar a significant number of African Americans from jobs at Dupont.

5. Most women have experienced months in which, when under great stress, their menstrual flow was delayed or failed to appear altogether. There is also the phenomenon of menstrual synchrony, in which girls/women who either live or spend lots of time together find their menstrual cycles synchronizing over a period of months. There is a distinct possibility that this shift toward coincidental timing may result from shared emotional states or environments.

6. The biomedical definition of menopause is not based on a woman's subjective experience of a gradual process of change in her particular menstrual pattern or on hot flashes in the continued presence of menstrual flow. Rather, biomedicine's determination is made retrospectively, after a woman has gone through twelve consecutive cycles without a menstrual flow. Kaufert (1988, 334) points out the methodological problems in this limited, nonsubjective definition, as "women may stop menstruating permanently, or for prolonged periods, for a variety of reasons other than pregnancy or menopause." Similarly, a definition based on cessation of the menses is limited to women of the western world who have limited childbearing, periods of lactation, and are of good nutritional status. For most other women in the world, amenorrhea is the norm and monthly menstrual flow is the exception. Many women pass from their last childbirth into menopause never having experienced intervening menstrual flow.

7. I would like to thank Jay Kaplan for encouraging me to write this piece and for listening to and questioning my ideas.

REFERENCES

Appell, Laura. 1988. Menstruation among the Rungus of Borneo: An Unmarked Category. In *Blood Magic: The Anthropology of Menstruation,* Thomas Buckley and Alma Gottlieb, eds., 94–112. Berkeley: University of California Press.

Buckley, Thomas, and Gottlieb, Anna (eds.) 1988. *Blood Magic: The Anthropology of Menstruation.* Berkeley: University of California Press.

Goodman, Madeleine J. 1982. A Critique of Menopause Research. In *Changing Perspectives on Menopause,* Ann M. Voda, Myra Dinnerstein, and Sheryl R. O'Donnell, eds., 273–88. Austin: University of Texas Press.

International Union, United Automobile, Aerospace and Agricultural Implement

Workers of America, UAW, et al. v. Johnson Controls, Inc. 1991. SC 113 L Ed 2d (1991) 158.

Kaufert, Patricia. 1980. The Menopausal Woman and Her Use of Health Services. *Maturitas* 2:191–206.

————. 1988. Menopause as Process or Event: The Creation of Definitions in Biomedicine. In *Biomedicine Examined,* Margaret Lock and D. R. Gordon, eds., 331–49. Norwell, Mass.: Kluwer.

Lander, Louise. 1988. *Images of Bleeding: Menstruation as Ideology.* New York: Orlando.

Lennon, Mary Clair. 1982. The Psychological Consequences of Menopause: The Importance of Timing of a Life Stage Event. *Journal of Health and Social Behavior* 23:353–66.

Lerman, Hannah. 1987. Personal correspondence.

Lichtman, Richard. 1981. Notes on Accumulation, Time and Aging. *Psychology and Social Theory* Spring/Summer 1:69–76.

McKinlay, John B.; McKinlay, Sonja M.; and Brambilla, Donald J. 1987a. Health Status and Utilization Behavior Associated with Menopause. *American Journal of Epidemiology* 125(1):110–21.

————. 1987b. The Relative Contributions of Endocrine Changes and Social Circumstances to Depression in Mid-Aged Women. *Journal of Health and Social Behavior* 28 (December):345–63.

McKinlay, Sonja M., and McKinlay, John B. 1973. Selected Studies of the Menopause. *Journal of Biosocial Science* 5:533–55.

Minow, Martha. 1990. *Making All the Difference: Inclusion, Exclusion, and American Law.* Ithaca, N.Y.: Cornell University Press.

Older Women's League. 1987. *The Picture of Health for Midlife and Older Women.* OWL, May.

Selfish Genes and Maternal Myths: A Look at Postmenopausal Pregnancy

Patricia Smith

"Menopause Found No Barrier to Pregnancy!" recent headlines announced. Reproductive technology is flying ahead at a dizzying pace, leaving moral discourse spinning in its wake. As science makes all things possible we must now decide which things are ethical or wise. In vitro fertilization is now readily available for an adequate price, as are "surrogate" mothers (that is, biological mothers who undergo pregnancy by contractual arrangement), and more recently, gestational mothers (that is, women who carry to term the transplanted embryo or fertilized ovum of another woman). And it turns out that a gestational mother (with further help from technology) can be postmenopausal. Age is now no barrier to "fertility" for women. Infertility is being brought under control—somebody's control. All this is, presumably, a good thing. The more control we have over our lives the better for all of us. And it is certain that women will never be free until we control our own reproductive capacities. So what is this nagging doubt in the back of my head—*are* we more in control? Am I among the "we" who are in control? If so, why do "we" (we, women) seem more out of control? And if not we women, who is in control?

A raft of problems arise with this latest medical triumph, and it would be wise to consider some of them before hailing it an unambiguous advance for women. How much are women (and men) being influenced by wizards of science playing games with people's bodies to solve abstract puzzles for the challenge of doing it, without considering its overall effect? How much are wizards of science being influenced by wizards of marketing and finance who know a good product when they see one? What is the function of money in this enterprise, and who is making funding decisions for this research? Is twenty-first-century medicine perpetuating nineteenth-century roles for women? It certainly wouldn't be the first time. If feminist historical research has demonstrated anything, it has shown clearly that the medical establishment, especially in the past two hundred years, has been extremely conservative about what it considers good for women, healthy for women, normal for women. Always it has assumed that the central (or only) function, fulfillment, and happiness of normal women is pregnancy, childbirth, and motherhood.

I would like to suggest that there are several good reasons to be skeptical about this latest advance of medical science, even beyond the obvious one, which is its dogged denial of the natural aging process as a reasonable and possibly even rewarding one. In addition to that, it is another instance of medical science addressing the problems of rich women for a fat fee, by glorifying pregnancy as the biological fulfillment of womanhood, and then providing the rich with special services they need in order to meet it. Furthermore, it perpetuates the old patriarchal tradition, which assumes the overriding significance of biological fatherhood as a right for men and a duty for women.

Medical Science and the Glorification of Pregnancy

The historical record of medical science's treatment of women is not one to inspire confidence. Let me mention just a few of the purported triumphs medical science has foisted on women in the past hundred years or so. During the late nineteenth century, while poor, working women were ignored, ladies of leisure were informed by the new experts of medical science that women are inherently sickly (Ehrenreich and English chap. 4). Women, it was thought, were simply by nature frail, and furthermore, their frailty, susceptibility to disease, and even personality disorders were all directly attributable to the power of their reproductive organs. This view was expressed, for example, by Dr. M. E. Dirix:

> Thus, women are treated for diseases of the stomach, liver, kidneys, heart, lungs, etc.; yet, in most instances, these diseases will be found on due investigation, to be, in reality, no diseases at all, but merely the sympathetic reactions or the symptoms of one disease, namely, a disease of the womb. (23–24)

Treatment for such disorders included application of leeches to the neck of the uterus, injections of various substances (such as milk or tea, even marshmallow) into the uterus, cauterization of the uterus (without anesthetic), removal of the clitoris, and removal of the ovaries (Barker-Benfield 122). By far the most popular cure for feminine disorders was the rest cure (very probably because it was relatively painless). The rest cure depended on total isolation and sensory deprivation techniques now identified with brainwashing. The patient was required to lie on her back in a dimly lit room for six weeks, concentrating exclusively on her proper function in life, namely, her reproductive function, with no visitors, conversation, or reading (no mental stimulation), only bland, soft food, and massages once a day. During this time she was literally commanded to health by her doctor. The effectiveness of this cure was thought to lie in the commanding, masculine force of the physician himself, along with the disengagement of the female brain from its war with the uterus.[1]

The war between the brain and the sexual organs (about which we have only recently forgotten) was longstanding and applied to men as well as women. But while men have always been advised to save their energy and strength for manly endeavors (which generally meant war or intellectual conquest), women were instructed to save themselves for their true vocation (which meant reproduction and domestic duties). Women have always been considered unfit for intellectual pursuits, but in certain periods of history (such as the late nineteenth and early twentieth centuries) doctors declared such activities not only futile but injurious to female health. Higher education would cause women's uteruses to wither, explained Dr. Edward H. Clarke, a Harvard professor whose best selling book, *Sex in Education, or a Fair Chance for the Girls,* went through seventeen editions within a few years. Following Clarke, medical research found that study caused pallor and delicate health in girls, as well as menstrual irregularity. (Bed rest was supposed to cure this.)[2] Higher education has also been held to cause (in women only) insanity (Bullough 323), sterility (Hall 632), the loss of lactation, (Hall 633), and even withering of the breasts.[3]

Doctors today no longer perform clitoridectomies or ovariotomies (at least not as cure-alls), and the application of leeches is long past. But let me mention a few more recent complaints. It has been estimated that half the hysterectomies performed in the United States in the past ten years were medically unnecessary (Ehrenreich and English 316). Debilitating total mastectomies are regularly performed when less intrusive remedies would be adequate (Love iv). The most common reason for performing Cesarean sections is convenience (Ehrenreich and English 316). The introduction of natural childbirth, much vaunted today, was opposed by doctors, as was the participation of fathers in the births of their children. Midwives have been virtually outlawed everywhere, thereby ensuring that all births will take place in (sterile but outrageously expensive) hospitals under the supervision of (expert but outrageously expensive) doctors, who are not necessarily giving us better treatment or advice than midwives did, or than clinics and nurse practitioners could for a fraction of the cost. As summed up by a recent writer:

> . . . routine use of anesthesia, and common resort to forceps, chemical induction of labor, and Caesarean sections turned out to be hazardous for mother and child, though convenient and probably gratifying to the physician. "Scientific" childbirth, for the sake of which the midwives had been outlawed, was revealed by the feminist critics as a drama of misogyny and greed. . . . Claiming the purity of science [the medical experts] had persisted in the commercialism inherent in a commoditized system of healing. . . . They turned out not to be scientists—for all their talk of data, laboratory findings, clinical trials—but apologists for the status quo. (Ehrenreich and English 316. See also O'Brien 1981)

Now, I don't mean to be cynical, and I do recognize that medical science has made revolutionary improvements in human life possible. But women do have reason to be a little circumspect before rushing down yet another primrose path with another "authority of medical science," especially when the effect is again to perpetuate women's traditional roles and again in a way that is lucrative to medical doctors.

By this I do not mean to suggest that there is no demand for this new service. Infertility, we are told, is on the rise among modern women (although oddly, not among poor women. It must be a disease of the rich, like gout).[4] There is no doubt that many career women are postponing childbearing until later in life only to discover that they are unable to conceive at thirty-five or forty or so. This is a serious problem, but these are not postmenopausal women. Most postmenopausal women are in their fifties. Now, why might a woman in her fifties decide that she wanted to experience pregnancy, and not as a fleeting whim, but as a sustained desire, strong enough to motivate her to undergo a very expensive and delicate medical procedure (ovum or embryo implantation) in order to spend nine months in a comparatively risky condition (as compared to pregnancy in younger women) culminating in the process of childbirth itself, which is extremely taxing even for a young and healthy woman? Just why would a mature woman want to do this?

Several putative reasons come to mind. It may be that she always wanted a child and was never able to have one before. She may have lost a child. Or her children may have grown up. She may be starting a new life with a new husband (say, after a divorce). All these reasons are understandable, but all could be accommodated more sensibly by adoption, especially, given the age of postmenopausal women, by the adoption of an older child.

So why embryo implantation rather than adoption? If the answer is that adoption is too difficult, or is unavailable, then there are two responses: (a) The couple (or single woman) needs to take a hard look at their (or her) ability to raise a child properly; (b) We all need to take a hard look at adoption policy in our society.

As to the first, prospective parents should ask themselves whether they are realistically healthy enough, strong enough, secure enough, and so on to take good care of a child for the next twenty years. People are not always very realistic about such matters. You may feel fine when you are fifty-five and acquire a newborn, but you will then be attending high school PTA meetings when you are seventy—a sobering thought if potential parents are willing to think it. It is interesting that in order to adopt a child you must qualify, that is, you must be able to persuade the authorities that you will be able to take care of the child. On the other hand, anyone at all can "grow their own" child through modern reproductive technology, and the only qualification you need is money. (Of course, if you are fertile you don't even need money.) So it may be that some older couples will have difficulty adopting a child, and there may be good reason for that. It hardly follows that if they do not qualify to adopt a child, they necessarily ought to have other means of obtaining one.

On the other hand, it hardly seems reasonable to rule out older people as a class from new parenthood. It is hardly humane or even sensible to make adoption so difficult that children in need cannot be placed with perfectly loving and decent parents simply because they do not fit a preconceived standardized mold that sets a single picture of an ideal family. Many combinations are reasonable. The object should be to bring people together, not to keep them apart. Our national adoption policy should reflect that rationale.

In addition, more mechanisms should be utilized to bring old and young people together who are not necessarily related, or closely related. You do not need to be a parent to share your life with a child. Aunts, uncles, grandparents, and friends can have an enormous effect on a child's life, and in today's busy world can be a real boon both to the child and the parents. Watching the blossoming of a child in whom you have invested time and love is always uniquely rewarding, whether it is your own child or someone else's. If none of these options appeal to you—if it is not enough to spend your time and energy on an adopted child or on someone else's child, perhaps you should examine your reasons for wanting a child. Perhaps you don't really want to spend time with a child. You just want to own one—but that issue will be addressed later.

In any case, a problem with adoption is not the only reason, or even the most likely reason for seeking postmenopausal pregnancy services. The difficulty of adoption is not the answer to our question in most cases. Since obtaining a child does not require going to the extreme of embryo implantation, there must be something in addition to a child that the postmenopausal woman or her husband wants. It is not just any child she wants. As commonly put, she wants a child "of her own," and somehow pregnancy provides that when adoption does not. Actually there are two possibilities here. She wants a child "of her own." Or her husband wants a child "of his own," and she wants to participate in that to the full extent of her ability. These are the two possibilities I now would like to discuss. Since, apparently, most people do not want "other people's children," or those they perceive to be other people's children, what makes a child "your own?"

The Selfish Gene, and a Plea for Adoption

Let's consider the father first. What makes the child "his own"? What makes the child really his? What makes him the real father? In our society and tradition (as well as nearly all others) the "real father" is the biological father—the man who contributes the genes.

Thus, one clear motivating factor which might encourage a woman to seek to attempt a postmenopausal pregnancy is a man who desires his own genetic offspring. By definition of the circumstances, genetic offspring are not a possibility for the postmenopausal woman. Presumably, she participates vicariously in the biological reproduction of her husband and another woman through the experience of pregnancy. It is a simulation of genetic reproduction for her. I shall have more to say about this in the next section, but for now the question is, Why is this important? From the point of view of biological reproduction, a postmenopausal woman is not reproducing herself or her family line, nor is she joining her family line with her mate's. So all that can be important from a biological point of view is the reproduction of the father's genetic line, his family, or perhaps by extension, his name.

Is this an objective or attitude that should be encouraged? I should like to argue that it is not, although I recognize that many people believe that as a basic drive the desire to reproduce is unavoidable. I am not convinced that it is unavoidable. It is certainly not universal, and certainly not without costs.

In *The Dialectic of Sex,* Shulamith Firestone argued that patriarchy itself is rooted in the biological inequality of the sexes. According to her, equality will only be possible when technology brings about a biological or reproductive revolution. Until women control their own reproduction, they will not change their fundamental condition no matter how much legal, political, or educational equality they acquire. Firestone envisioned a day when children could be conceived and gestated ex utero, a time when the physical involvement of women in the production of children would be analogous to that of men, freeing women to pursue any of life's callings on an equal footing with men. For Firestone, biological motherhood was (and is) an anchor for women, or a ball and chain from which they can be released only by a liberating technology.

Beyond this source of inevitable sex inequality, however, Firestone saw biological parenthood as a source of further evils, especially the vice of possessiveness, which generates envy, hostility, and inequality among classes and races as well as between the sexes. Why, she asked, do men wish to amass property to bequeath to their children and thus withhold it from all others? As she saw it, the vice of possessiveness, the favoring of one's own child as the product of one's own seed, is the major source of division and hierarchy which must be overcome if the future is to be better than the past.

Furthermore, she argued, in the current (patriarchal) social structure, people too often desire children for the wrong reasons. In a patriarchal system, for a man, a child is an ego extension, a way to immortalize himself: his name, his property, his business, his estate, his genetic line; for a woman, a child is a justification of her (dependent) existence, her reason for living as she does. Too often, it is not a genuine liking of children, Firestone suggests, that motivates reproduction, but instead a displacement of ego-extension needs. This sort of motivation can be destructive both for parents and children.

Thus, for Firestone, the human focus on biological offspring is the most fundamental source of inequality between the sexes, of hierarchical class systems, of economic inequality, and of some of the most destructive vices to which human beings succumb. As a result, she concluded that the biological family (the focus on genetic offspring) should be replaced with a more broadly sympathetic unit when technology makes such an alternative possible.

Firestone's thesis has been attacked (and defended) for twenty years by both feminists and others, but her ideas are not easily dismissed. Feminists generally agree with Firestone that biological inequality produced patriarchy with all its attendant disadvantages for women; but many disagree that the only way out is to eliminate biological inequality through technology. First, some have argued that biological motherhood is not necessarily limiting. It is not a disability, but an ability. Adrienne Rich, for example, has argued that it is not pregnancy and motherhood itself that oppresses women, but the fact that women are not themselves in control of these conditions. We do not know what pregnancy and birth would be like in a nonpatriarchal setting in which women could experience biological motherhood on their own terms. Thus, she urges, women should not give up on biological motherhood without ever having been in charge of it.

Other feminists focus strongly on the dangers of technology and fault Firestone for her uncritical acceptance of it. Mary O'Brien, for example, claims that while the process of reproduction has been the source of women's oppression, it is also the ground of their liberation. All the advances in technology have not broken male control over female fertility, O'Brien observes. On the contrary, female fertility has been industrialized, legalized, and "medicalized," keeping it in the hands of the conservative male establishment. Opposition to midwives and nurse practitioners, free-standing abortion clinics, home birthing, and self-administered artificial insemination are examples of resistance to low-tech procedures over which women could exert more control. We should be wary of new high-tech procedures, O'Brien warns, for they may be used not to liberate women, but to gain further control over them.

Gena Corea has extended this argument, noting that modern technology has broken the female reproductive process into even smaller pieces, thus reducing the power of the mother and her claim to the child.[5] All these arguments give one pause about Firestone's uncritical acceptance of modern reproductive technology; but in fact none of them really challenge her basic points that biological inequality under patriarchy maintains sex inequality, class inequality, and the vice of possessiveness. On the contrary, they seem to support such claims. And other philosophers have inadvertently supported these views in an interesting way (perhaps the strongest way) by assuming that they are true. Particularly, libertarians and economic theorists have argued that redistribution of wealth schemes are and will always be ineffective or wrong (or both) because individuals will always find ways to favor their own children. F. A. von Hayek, for example, argued that it is not the structure of the economy which makes some classes disadvantaged and others advantaged, but the structure of families. The only way to eliminate inequality, he claimed, would be to eliminate families (von Hayek chap. 6). That is exactly what Firestone argued.

The difference between the two is that Firestone thought the logical conclusion was to eliminate families (at least in their present form); von Hayek thought the logical conclusion was to accept inequality as inevitable. And that is the most powerful argument against Firestone (not the feminist quibbles which actually add to her critique rather than diminish it). Furthermore, the objection of impossibility is also the common-sense response one would receive from the man on the street, and very probably from the woman on the street as well. The objection goes like this: Firestone may rail against the biological family all she likes, and even demonstrate that it causes all sorts of evils, but it is impossible to eliminate it. Human beings have a natural drive to reproduce themselves biologically. Asking them not to do so is like asking them not to eat. To try to subvert biological reproduction is a foolish and futile project because the sex drive is a fundamental and unalterable human need. So Firestone's radical suggestions are useless and so are the more moderate suggestions that older people should redirect their energies to adopting children and sharing in the lives of other people's children.

In answer to this common-sense objection I would suggest first that while there certainly is a biological sex drive, the drive is for sex and not for reproduction. I am not suggesting that there is no drive for reproduction whatsoever; but in terms of a basic drive that corresponds in some way to instinctual drives in animals, the drive is for sexual interaction. It is coincidental (from the viewpoint of human psychology or desire) that it sometimes results in reproduction. In our inimitable human way we have abstracted sexuality from reproduction as such and put it to all sorts of other uses. Sexual intercourse is used by human beings for any number of purposes including, but not limited to, the expression of love, hate, sympathy, domination, unification, masochism, sadism, companionship, playfulness, support, and entrapment. Reproduction is simply one purpose among many for which it is used, and not even (I would suggest) the primary one. At least, enormous energy and ingenuity have been expended to reliably (or even unreliably) ensure that sexual intercourse will not result in reproduction. And that enterprise has increased with the impracticality of having children in an overpopulated world and a highly technical and urban environment.

If reproduction itself is a basic drive, it has diminished in interesting ways in the past one hundred years or so. Given the falling birth rates, it would appear that human beings in advanced industrialized countries no longer have this urge more often than once or twice in a lifetime. Or if they do feel it more often than that, it must not be so strong an urge that they cannot fairly easily resist it. On the other hand, in other countries where education and birth control are not as readily available, or where the economy is still agrarian, the urge seems to have remained strong. Now, if this is a basic human drive, why would the strength of its existence vary from place to place or time to time? Furthermore, what kind of a basic drive is it that is commonly not experienced more than once or twice in a lifetime?

Clearly, the basic drive is the drive for sex. That has remained constant over time and place. And it certainly is commonly experienced more than once or twice in a lifetime. But, as I have mentioned, the sex drive has been separated from the drive to reproduce (if there is one) in human beings.

Nevertheless, it may be objected that even if people do not want to have children as often as they have sex, they still do want to have children. Furthermore, they want to have children of "their own," that is, their own biological offspring.

That may be true—indeed it is true—but that does not make it a basic drive, and it certainly does not make it an unalterable basic drive. It could as easily be the product of socialization and norm. It certainly is not universal; that is, not all people care about it. Not all men want children at all, let alone feel driven to reproduce. Indeed, as social pressure slackens and diverse individual lifestyles become more accepted, more couples are choosing not to have children. I assume that men who do not want children are still normal. So what does the biological claim amount to? We have at this point in time very little evidence for the continued existence of human biological instincts as opposed to social construction and adaptation. Who knows whether we have any instincts at all any more—especially for something as complicated as a felt need to reproduce one's genetic line?

And some modern men themselves are finding reason to have second thoughts about the genetic model of paternity or child ownership. With divorces and single parenthood, family relations can be complex today. Recently a young man who had married a woman with a baby from a previous relationship told me that he resented references to the child's biological father (whom the child never saw) as the "real" father. "I'm the real father," he told me. "I fed her her bottle at 2:00 in the morning. I held her when she was sick. I taught her her ABCs. I bring home a paycheck every week and make sure she eats right. I'm the one she comes to when she needs something. I'm the one she runs to hug every day after work. She calls *me* Daddy. And she's *mine*."

Personally, I think he is right. After all, she will most likely have his values, his thoughts, his assumptions, even his mannerisms, his expressions, his sense of humor. She will be influenced by his attitudes, his reasoning, his standards, and his expectations. Surely it is the forming of a mind and a character that makes a child "your own." It is the sharing of life through good times and bad that forms a bond between parent and child. The real father is the one who spends time and energy and love. The real father is the man who shares his life, who remains committed, who is there—not always physically there, perhaps—but there.

This is admittedly a messy notion of paternity. Lawyers would hate it because it would produce a lot of unclear cases. In real life, of course, there *are* a lot of unclear cases. "Good Heavens!" any good lawyer would say, "On this definition a child could wind up with two or three fathers (or mothers)!" How terrible. Would it be so debilitating for a child to know that more than one man loves her like a father? And if the law declares it not so, will that make it not so? I think the law should have to face the messy cases of real life and not make them clear by stipulative definition. Anyway, this messy notion of paternity is no worse than the one we have now which enables the law to take a child away from a man who cares for her and give her to one who does not. But my concern here is not with legal definitions (although I wouldn't mind defending this view in another paper), but with social attitudes, which are really much more important. The question I asked is, What makes a man's child "his own"? and the unstated question implicit in the other is, Why should the answer be his genes?

The trouble with prevalent social attitudes today is that they carry on unreflectively the old patriarchal glorification of the "seed" that incorporates a notion of children as property, women as caretakers, and biology as destiny. This idea was never very good, even in its heyday, and it is certainly outdated now. It was once considered a sign of manhood to produce many children. Not to raise, or feed, or care for, or love many children—just to produce many children. It was important to plant a lot of seed, and children were supposed to grow up somehow on their own, like plants. That is part of the glorification of the seed. Your children are supposed to grow up like you because they came from your seed. Biology is destiny. Of course, that is ludicrous as applied to human beings. Yet our history is replete with amazing legends and myths of men running around planting seed, moving on to new adventures, and returning in twenty years or so to see how things came out. And did things come out well? Of course they did. Blood tells. It is also the case that the little woman stayed home faithfully all that time to see to it that sonny came out like his dad. Or maybe it was a kindly elf who took care of him. Or even a pack of wolves. In any case the moral of the story is that it matters not at all how you are raised or by whom, least of all by your own father, whose presence is completely inessential because, in the end, breeding counts. If you have prince genes, you're a prince. That in itself makes you a prince, and those qualities will show up sooner or later no matter what your life has been like. That story was still being propagated in *Star Wars,* one of the best sellers of the past decade.

In my opinion, as romantic as it is, as exciting as it is, as convenient as it is for irresponsible men, this whole complex of ideas needs to be ditched. And we have made some progress in this direction. Legally, a sperm donor has no claim whatsoever to any resulting child. Rationally, we no longer think that it makes no difference whether a father is present in the raising of his children. But the romantic idea of the significance of the seed hangs on. It is very hard to fight a romantic idea because such ideas are not rational. They lay no claim to rationality, so rational argument cannot dislodge them. What we need are new stories with different morals and, most of all, with different heroes. That will not be easy. But it will be worth it.

But perhaps this is too one-sided, and anyway what does it prove? It shows that some men develop the same love for an adopted child as anyone could have for a child that is genetically connected to him. In fact, examples of this are plentiful among both adoptive fathers and adoptive mothers. Genetic connection is not necessary for bonding. Nor is it sufficient. It is well known that a fair number of men (and some women) produce children and walk away forever. The truth is that very few princes who sowed their seed ever checked back to see how anybody was doing. Bastards were on their own. The patriarchal legend of the significance of the seed never seemed to encourage responsibility among the sowers of seed for the products of their planting. So nothing follows from genetic connection one way or the other.

Having said that, it is nevertheless clear that biological connection is important to many people. This could be due to many factors, several of which I have already mentioned. Let's consider further the patriarchal tradition. Until about the fourteenth century it was not known that there is a female seed. Women were seen as containers or vessels within which the male seed developed. For men, this provided a kind of immortality. A man's line could be traced through his name (passed down from father to son), his estate (also retained by male children, especially the first born), and his seed (or his blood, it was thought—those genetic characteristics that he managed to transfer to his offspring, which we now know are minimal by the third generation if not before). A man's body may disintegrate after he dies but his name, his property, and his characteristics, it was thought, could be perpetuated through his children. So a man's child, especially his son, was like a piece of himself or an extension of himself. He might hope to accomplish through his son what he couldn't manage to do himself. Perhaps he didn't go to college, but his son would. He wasn't a professional man, but his son would be. Or he might perpetuate his business or estate. His son might take over the family farm or the family business or follow his trade. So a man could dream that his projects need not die with him, for they could be carried on by his sons.

And even if such plans as these did not materialize, just having someone to carry on your name and seed continues to be important to some men even today. Just recently it was reported that some soldiers before shipping out to the Middle East conflict, stopped off at sperm banks, so that their wives could attempt to perpetuate their names or blood lines or ensure their immortality in case they did not return.

Nor do these desires necessarily diminish with age. It is not rare for a man in his fifties or sixties, especially one who remarries to a younger woman, to produce children, a second family. It can be a way of starting over.

But let's examine all this. What does it presuppose? To my mind it assumes just the kind of attitude that I was condemning. The young soldiers are assuming that their children can be raised without them and still be theirs. Their mother will take care of them faithfully, instilling all the values and habits (and memories?) that the father would have wanted his children to have. She will carry out his program. He just has to lay down the law, not carry it out. He just provides the seed. Somebody else is the gardener.

That is also, by and large, what the older man assumes. He can have a child at sixty because someone else will be the primary caretaker. This is what Firestone was condemning: having children not because you like children, not because you plan to spend your life with them, but as ego extensions, as sources of immortality. Being the source of your father's immortality and the caretaker of his dreams can be very burdensome. How many children have been pushed into careers because a parent always wanted to do it? The lives of sons were once literally ruled by the ambitions of their fathers. This is not as true today because fathers simply do not have as much control; but the attitude is still oppressive for children.

Having said all this, it is still clear that a great many people do not have children for the wrong reasons, and the reasons they have them may be rather amorphous. I suspect that the right reasons are something like the desire to make a home, a family, and a future—a commitment to a certain sort of life. And mixed in with all that is the inarticulate sense that somehow your biological children are reproductions of yourself or the person you love. (It is not always yourself that you want to reproduce.) This is mostly mythology, of course. For the most part, our children are not much like us beyond their socialization. But there will usually be a trait or two that enable you to say, "Oh, yes, she has her father's eyes," or feet, or temper, or whatever, and that is enough to perpetuate the myth. Sometimes, in fact, there is a striking resemblance, but even when there is, if we are truthful, we must admit that even a son who looks just like his father is not a reproduction of his father. There will be a lot about him that is not like his father at all. Human beings are complex and individual. We pretend that we can reproduce ourselves, but in fact we cannot. All we can reproduce is the species.

Wouldn't it be better to face it? Wouldn't it be better to recognize that even if biological parenthood is the norm (and I am not arguing that it ought not to be) it doesn't provide anything other than a child?

It does not make you immortal. Genetic transferral dissipates within a few generations. You cannot select what gets transferred anyway, so you are just as likely to "bequeath" your big nose or your fallen arches or your diabetes as you are any good quality you might like to immortalize. More to the point, what is really important about you—your character, your beliefs, your ideals, your wit, your personality—the whole complex that makes up the real *you* cannot be transferred genetically. A biological child cannot make you immortal.

And it cannot make you a "real man" either. I confess that I do not know what makes a man "real" (whatever that means), but it can't be that. Biological reproduction simply cannot be the standard of manhood. It would not distinguish a man from an elephant or a walrus. Anyway, I understand that the real pros at reproduction are rats and cockroaches. There has to be a better standard. Biological reproduction cannot make you a real man.

I have already discussed what makes a man a real father, and it has nothing to do with genes. It has to do with character and commitment.

So what is so significant about biological paternity? Is it convenient?

Yes. Is it significant? No. Fatherhood, however, is a different story. Fatherhood is very significant. It is a uniquely human endeavor. It is among the highest of callings. And it enlists the best qualities a man can summon for one of the noblest and most crucial of causes, the raising of a child, who is not a reproduction of himself, but who is part of a new generation, and therefore the only possible hope for the future. Doing that job well will necessarily require all your heart and all your mind, but not necessarily any of your genes. When men finally learn this, everyone will be better off.

Childbirth as the Fulfillment of Womanhood

The most disturbing feature of the promotion of postmenopausal pregnancy is not its presumption of the primacy of the biological offspring of men. Nor is it even its head-in-the-sand assumption that people do not age, and so it is perfectly fine to take on a heavy twenty-year obligation, to make someone else dependent on you, when you are heading for social security. I can even live with the fact that it is yet another instance of medical science conveniently solving a problem of the rich for a conveniently large fee.

The really disturbing feature of the very idea of postmenopausal pregnancy is that the only clear justification for it is that it is somehow fulfilling for women. It resurrects the old idea that somehow a woman hasn't really achieved womanhood; she hasn't really lived; she hasn't been fulfilled until she has been pregnant. Postmenopausal pregnancy serves no other clear purpose. Every other objective could be achieved more easily and safely by other means. The argument must be that the very experience of pregnancy and childbirth is intrinsically rewarding (or that a woman is obligated to do it for her husband, which is just as bad). Indeed, so rewarding, so essential to well-being and self-respect is this experience for a woman that it is worth producing a child that she will be caring for in her sixties and seventies.

Recently it was reported that seven women in or past menopause became pregnant with eggs donated by younger women and fertilized with their husbands' sperm. Among them was a woman who had undergone various fertility treatments for an entire decade. Her pregnancy ended in the tragedy of stillbirth, but she is determined to try again (Goodman).

I know nothing else about this woman, so I will not presume to discuss her particular case except to express my sincere sympathy. Cases like hers, however, exemplify the enormous pressure many women feel to bear children. Why? Is the experience of pregnancy and childbirth so intrinsically rewarding that resorting at the age of fifty to the implantation of another woman's ovum is generally understandable and sane? What picture of the basic role, identity, and function of women is implied in such an attitude? Are we not "real women" if we haven't been pregnant? Are we not "real mothers" unless we ourselves give birth?

Indeed, just such views and related ones have been put forward for centuries as the standard of normalcy for women. The analogue of the male seed is the female flowerpot. Pregnancy makes the child "her own." The "real" mother gives birth to the child.[6]

Women have always been conditioned to view their destiny and fulfillment as motherhood. Throughout the ages, myths and ballads, novels and operas have extolled the virtues of motherhood as the destiny of womankind and deplored the tragedy of the woman gone astray from her natural mission. The entire force of law, politics, culture, art, morality, custom, and medical science combined to ensure that few would stray from the maternal path. Even in the past 150 years when dissatisfaction with the exclusive role of mothering has become ever more difficult to quell, the experts have staunchly defended motherhood as the only source of genuine fulfillment for normal women.

Many of the cures I listed in the first section were intended to reconcile the "abnormal" (that is, the dissatisfied) woman to her mission in life, namely, her reproductive function. In case the discussion there left you with the impression that the psychoanalytic function of gynecology was an early phase of medicine that died out at the turn of the century, consider this advice to gynecologists, offered in 1962:

> We feel this discipline [gynecology] should embrace those disturbances in function or structure of any part of the female organism that influence or are affected by the performance of the reproductive system. We are impressed in particular with the dictum that much of the physical and mental ill health of the individual woman can be properly understood *only* in light of her conscious or unconscious acceptance of her *feminine role*. (Sturgis xiv; emphasis added)

It sounds a lot like the study in 1906, doesn't it? Women are not healthy unless they want to be mothers. According to one historian, gynecologists in the 1950s and 1960s began to view the following conditions as resulting from "incomplete feminization": menstrual pain or irregularity, excessive pain in labor, infertility, miscarriage, premature birth, excessive nausea in pregnancy, toxemia, complications of labor, and pelvic pain (e.g., in Sturgis; see Osofsky 146). Thus, once again it became the gynecologists' role to help every woman adjust to her true nature and, most of all, not let her allegiance to her brain outweigh her allegiance to her uterus. Nor were gynecologists alone in this mission. Psychiatrists were also up to the task, enlisting other doctors as well to the cause of keeping women in line with their true needs, which meant the eradication of the maladjustment of "rejection of femininity."[7]

Of course, for Freudians, pregnancy was the answer to penis envy, a way for a woman to overcome her own long-resented "castration," enabling her to accept her femininity. Accepting femininity has been terribly important to Freudians (almost as important as it has been to gynecologists). Erik Erikson, for example, theorized that because of their biology women (or girls) were concerned with inner space (like the inside of building) and with procreation. While the penis is apparent and present, by contrast the womb is apparently absent, symbolizing a lack and thus a need in women. Pregnancy, then, constitutes fulfillment (almost literally) while childlessness stands for emptiness and despair (Erikson 582–606).

Another influential psychoanalyst of about the same period, Helene Deutsch, described the *Psychology of Women* as a balance of passivity, masochism, and narcissism (her paradigm of a normal woman). A woman's masochism consisted in an attraction to experiences like childbirth and sexual intercourse which mix pleasure with pain. (According to her, orgasm is a lot like labor. That's what she says!) Woman's passivity was central to her role in intercourse and in life. If a woman was too aggressive or too intellectual, she was "rejecting her femininity." The important thing for a normal woman was to maintain balance among her three dominant characteristics, and the best way to do that was (guess what) by recourse to frequent pregnancy, first, as a hedge against the inevitable loss of one's child (they do grow up), and second, as a means of disciplining one's selfish desires to narcissism or away from passivity, and thus, femininity.[8]

In the 1950s and 1960s there was apparently a great rash of "rejection of femininity." Therapists and gynecologists seemed to find it everywhere.[9] Nor were doctors and analysts alone in keeping women on course to their great mission and true needs. Novelists and poets, songwriters and journalists were all doing their bit to romanticize and see to the perpetuation of motherhood as the central role and fulfillment of women (although by this time the forces were no longer unified).[10]

Furthermore, there are feminists who celebrate pregnancy and birthing as unique sources of power and liberation for women (see, e.g., Rich), and who define a mother in terms of pregnancy and birth as well as childrearing. For such feminists a "real mother" understands the hardship and magic of carrying a child within her for nine months, knows the pain and exhilaration of giving birth and the tranquility of suckling a baby (e.g., Donchin 131). With so much adulation and guidance, it is hardly any wonder if many women still see pregnancy as the glorious fulfillment of womanhood.

This view was perfectly understandable a hundred years ago. For centuries every woman's life and well-being, her purpose for existing, as well as her source of security were tied up in her production of children. Women were mothers. That was their identity. That was their role. That was the only purpose and function they had. Thus, the sad picture of the childless woman in previous centuries was truly a picture of tragedy. The childless woman was faced with an empty life, quite literally, a life without purpose, and possibly a life without value. She would be a burden. The best she could do was help out others, perhaps, do the spinning. Small wonder that pregnancy was viewed as fulfillment. Pregnancy was the promise of a child, a future, a purpose, a place in the world order. But surely it is not hard to see that while pregnancy was (and is) a symbol and a promise, it was not pregnancy itself which was important. It was the child that was important. The only reason pregnancy was important for a woman was (a) it was the only way to get (or rather produce) a child, and (b) producing a child was the only reason for a woman to exist. One hundred years ago all that made sense. It may not have been fair; it certainly was not equal treatment, but it made perfectly good sense. In today's world, however, there are two major problems with this kind of thinking, namely both *a* and *b* are now false.

Consider *b*. Producing a child was once the only reason for a woman to exist. But women no longer live such restricted lives. This has not been true for very long, and it still is not true in many places. Perhaps we should remember that when we start to get impatient. Women in general have only been free to pursue careers for two generations at most, but great changes have taken place in that time. Particularly two changes.

First, a woman today can be entirely independent. She may not want to be, but she can be. She need not marry, let alone bear children, in order to live. She can be economically self-sufficient and autonomous.

Second, she can pursue virtually any calling or career. Thus, a woman is now free to determine her own goals and purposes, set by her own decisions. It may not be easy, but it is possible, and more importantly, it is thinkable. When my grandmother was growing up, what I am doing now was unthinkable for an ordinary woman. The average person simply could not imagine it. It was so extraordinary as to be farfetched. It was still pretty farfetched when my mother was growing up. But now it is both thinkable and possible, and the more women do it, the more thinkable and possible and ordinary and normal it will become.

So it now makes no sense to talk about *the* function of women—*the* reason for women's existence as a class—*the* purpose of womankind. There is no more purpose of womankind than there is a purpose of mankind. Now that both men and women are free, there are only many purposes and many people to pursue them. So *b* is false.

At the same time, it is worth remembering that all this is new, and social change progresses unevenly. It is thus understandable that many women still think of their only purpose in life as motherhood. For these women infertility may be a great tragedy, or they may find adoption a reasonable alternative. That brings me to a consideration of *a*.

According to tradition—the received wisdom—pregnancy is the only means to motherhood. Pregnancy—the production of a child—is the meaning of motherhood and the fulfillment and destiny of women. "Real women" are mothers and "real mothers" give birth. It is that set of ideas that is my greatest concern, and it is that set of ideas which is most closely associated with the notion of postmenopausal pregnancy. The whole situation reflects the desperation of the childless woman of a century ago.

I am not suggesting that every woman who undergoes this procedure is desperate. I am concerned over those who are, and I am concerned about a new technology that suggests once again that the fulfillment of women is pregnancy, because it encourages just that sort of desperation. Women are encouraged to feel unfulfilled if they haven't experienced pregnancy. It suggests that there is something terribly important about the experience of pregnancy itself.

But why? What is important about pregnancy in and of itself—the experience of pregnancy? Does it make women better mothers? Or better human beings? Does it make them loving, kind, nurturing, supportive?

That in fact has been suggested. It has even been suggested by feminists.[11] But it is clearly false. A fair number of women give birth to children whom they subsequently neglect or abuse. Giving birth is no guarantee of subsequent good motherhood. None whatever. Quite the contrary. Babies are more likely to be guaranteed a good home with adoptive mothers than with birth mothers.

The experience of pregnancy and childbirth may be profound, but it does not change a woman's personality. It is not mind altering. At least it didn't change any woman I have ever known. Mothers, like all other human beings, vary widely in their personalities and characters. Some are warm and loving. Some are cold and distant. Some are temperamental and abusive, and so on. However a woman was before she got pregnant is very probably how she will be after she gives birth (except that she will be more tired). Pregnancy does not make a woman loving and patient if she was not so before. Child care might, especially under the right conditions and over time, but that does not require pregnancy.

Does pregnancy make a woman mature? Clearly not, since there are many highly immature mothers. I strongly suspect that the experience of pregnancy and childbirth in and of itself has very little long-term effect on the personality or character of most women. (Again, taking responsibility for the child might, but that does not require pregnancy.) Furthermore, if pregnancy does change a woman, there is no evidence that it changes her for the better. Why should it? The mental experience may be happy—assuming that a woman is happy about it. But the physical experience on the whole is either tedious or traumatic. What do you suppose it does for a rape victim? Does it improve her character?

It is sometimes suggested that, having gone through the suffering of nine long months of pregnancy and the trauma and pain of childbirth, a woman is more committed to her child, more connected, even less individual. She sees herself as intrinsically related to her child in a way that no one else can quite duplicate. That is the special bond that pregnancy provides. Being literally connected to her child forms a bond that is particularly powerful and that is what makes her a better mother or gives her special insight into her child's needs.

There are actually several points combined in this view. First, we simply have no evidence that suffering makes people better. In fact, we have more evidence that it makes people neurotic. It may make some people sympathetic to the suffering of others, but it hardens most people. It may make some people strong. It clearly destroys others. And even if it makes some people strong, that does not make them good. Some very strong people are very nasty. For that matter, some very strong mothers are very nasty.

I once knew a woman who regularly reminded her children (often in my presence, or anyone else's) how much she had suffered giving birth to them, how much she had given up for them, and how much they consequently owed her in return—namely, everything. They owed her their lives, she said. She was an ordinary housewife. I don't know why she thought her suffering was so special. Nor is it clear to me what she gave up. But it is clear to me that suffering did not improve her character. And I see no reason to assume without evidence that it is generally good for people—even mothers. So much for suffering.

The second suggestion is that because of their literal connection during pregnancy, women have special (instinctive) insight into the needs of babies. This is also completely false and one of the most pernicious rumors circulated by the patriarchal tradition. I have heard many men and women make this claim, and of course it is terribly convenient for men who don't want to get up and see what is wrong with the baby, or take responsibility for it, or learn how to take care of it.

This is analogous to the attitude that many women have about cars, and thus generates an analogous stereotype. "Oh, I just don't understand cars," they claim. "I just don't have any aptitude for it." But a woman who has total responsibility for herself and must supply her own transportation will quickly develop such an aptitude. All you have to do is run your car without oil once. After you find that you have to buy yourself a new car as the price of your lack of aptitude, you will find that you can remember things like tune-ups and oil changes just fine. Most women who don't learn to do this, don't learn to do it because they assume that it is someone else's job, usually their husband's. He pays attention to that kind of thing. It is a matter of delegating responsibility. You delegate responsibility to someone else and then put the whole matter out of your mind. You never think about it; you never pay attention to it; so you never learn how to deal with it. That is exactly the same way many men are with babies.

Women have the same power of deduction and induction that men have, and this is true whether they have ever been pregnant or not. Any of us can look at a problem and run through the alternatives which might solve it, until we find the best solution. The more experienced you are in any given area, the quicker and more accurate you are likely to be at solving problems within it. The only reason that women appear to have instincts about caring for babies is that girls tend to be channeled into child care long before they are adults, and boys tend not to be.

I am a normal woman (I think); at least I am as strongly tied to my children as anyone. But when I had my first baby (about which I was very gung ho, by the way—natural childbirth and all that goes with it), I discovered that I had *no* idea how to take care of it. I didn't know why it was crying any more than anyone else did. And that is because I was a tomboy. I never took care of babies as a girl, or watched anybody else do it, or thought about doing it. So when it came time to do it I didn't know how. But I learned very quickly, as anyone can who is interested and assumes responsibility for it.[12] I can assure you that women who have no previous experience with babies will have no informative "instincts" about them either. No innate knowledge about how to take care of babies is generated simply from the experience of being pregnant.

The third suggestion is that either the suffering or the connectedness of pregnancy makes women more committed or loyal to their children. We do not have any evidence for this either, although it is a more complex and interesting claim than the other two, and not as obviously false. It is factually true that very few women abandon their children. Whatever their faults otherwise—they may not be loving, or kind, or consistent, or even-tempered, but very few women simply leave home. And that is not true of men. A fair number of men produce children and walk away. So what is the most reasonable explanation?

I do not think that the most reasonable explanation is the biological one. I do think that it may be reasonable to suppose that some notion of instinct and pregnancy do play a part, but not in the way that is commonly suggested, namely, that women have instincts that men do not have. Probably all human beings have an instinct for survival, and perhaps some sort of instinctive respect for life. Even if they do, however, it is not instinct which is different in men and women, but social conditioning and circumstances.[13]

If a man were confronted directly with a helpless infant (suppose he tripped over one out in the woods, or discovered a foundling on his front porch), he would not just keep walking, or throw it in the trash, any more than a woman would. What he would do, probably, is find someone else to take care of it. He would delegate it. But suppose he lived in some very remote area? Suppose that there were no one else to care for the infant? I submit that in a case like that most men (a very high percentage) would keep the baby, would try to take care of it one way or another. If human beings have any instincts at all, one of them must be a kind of reverence for human life as such. Now, we manage to warp and twist and distort that reverence in all sorts of amazing ways. We have managed to exclude from the human race whole classes, races, and nationalities. But even as we engage in these distortions, it remains very difficult for almost any human being to ignore a helpless infant if directly confronted. I do not know whether it explains anything to construe that as instinct; but whatever it is, both men and women have it generally, and neither sex has it universally.

What certainly is different between men and women are their circumstances, and a big part of that difference is due to pregnancy. In my view, the really significant thing about pregnancy is that at the end of it you are directly confronted with a helpless infant who is entirely dependent on you for its life. Now combine this with social conditioning. Since pregnancy always has been exclusively a capacity of women we have had plenty of time to develop the socially useful idea that it is biologically impossible for a woman to leave her child. It was probably very important for women to believe that at one time, and it is probably true for any human being faced with leaving an infant to die. But it is no longer true that an infant will die if a mother decides not to keep it. Yet the social conditioning hangs on. What kind of a woman are you if you can leave your child? You are a biological deviant, something like a sociopath. You lack some crucial humanizing feature. You are a moral monster or at least seriously deficient. Women are conditioned to believe that any woman who can leave her child with someone else is a moral defective. I have even heard such criticisms (even self-criticism) applied to working mothers who leave their children in child-care centers. It is unforgivably selfish, irretrievably irresponsible. Much worse that any thing a man could ever do. A cruel or unfeeling mother is the most evil creature the human imagination can invent. With such strong conditioning it should not be surprising that most women have a very difficult time giving up their children for adoption, even when they know, rationally, that it would be best for the child. What kind of a woman is she if she can do it? Men are not faced with social conditioning or circumstances of this sort.

As I said, it is probably exceedingly difficult (although I would not say biologically impossible) for almost any human being to abandon a totally helpless infant. But the fact is, all infants come into the world directly connected to a mother, so men are rarely confronted with a helpless infant unattended by someone else. Consider the differences in the circumstances of men and women. A woman is necessarily confronted with her child (and is additionally conditioned to keep it). A man can initiate a pregnancy and be gone for many months before an infant ever appears. We may say that some men produce children and then just walk away; but who did they walk away from? Not the child, but the mother. And even when a man walks away from both mother and child, he is not leaving a child to die. He is leaving the child with its mother, which tradition and common wisdom all tell him is the person best suited to take care of it anyway.

I am not suggesting that this is acceptable, or even excusable. I am suggesting that social conditioning, based on the unsupported assumption that women, but not men, are biologically incapable of leaving their children, enforces a norm that may make women more responsible but certainly encourages men to be less so. There is no way to confirm or refute the biological claim. It is not clear that it does anything that could not be accomplished better in other ways. And its side effects are terrible. So why assume it?

The values associated with motherhood—commitment, nurturance, security, goodness, support, comfort, love, loyalty—are needed throughout the world. They are needed, it has often been said, to preserve humanity from the dehumanizing effects of capitalism, or the trials of public life. We all need a home, a safe haven, and typically, mother has kept the home fires burning.

But to tie those values to the experience of pregnancy sharply limits them and thus makes them tenuous as human values. If human beings cannot achieve this ultimately virtuous state without going through some magical transformation only accomplished through the wonder and trauma of pregnancy and childbirth, then the world is in serious trouble. It follows that no childless women, even adoptive mothers, and no men at all can hope to achieve the ultimate state of love achieved by birth mothers. But that is clearly false. Most of us know this if we reflect on people we know. Perhaps some do not know it because they have been deprived of the best experiences life has to offer. I happened to know that it was false the first time I heard it suggested, because I happen to know that no one can love more than my father loves me. I really don't think that has anything to do with his genes. I can't prove it, of course. But I think it has to do with who he is, and who I am, and something or other that we have shared for long enough that it can't go away, ever.

My mother and father are both very loving and committed parents. They are a team. They love each other, and they love their children. They are good at it. Their commitment is strong and inclusive. But neither one of them ever suggested or seemed to think that any one person had a monopoly on the ability to love or be committed. And I don't see why it would be reasonable, helpful, or accurate to suppose that anyone does—even mothers who have gone through pregnancy.

So, what is the great value of pregnancy in and of itself? The final claim many people make is that women need it (e.g., Erikson; and Deutsch, among others too numerous to mention). (That is certainly what the Freudians think.) We, women, need to be pregnant in order to be fulfilled, to overcome our penis envy. Ignoring all that, what exactly is fulfilling about pregnancy? Having been pregnant myself several times, you would think that I would be able to answer that question right off; but in all honesty "fulfilling" is not a word that I would have chosen to describe pregnancy itself. However, many women do—so what does that mean? "Fulfilling" as an adverb, means "satisfying or gratifying." This is actually a very simple notion of "fulfilling" that could apply to any number of things. Some women find social work fulfilling. Some find golf fulfilling. Some find needlepoint fulfilling. Others find fulfillment in the practice of law. Any number of things can be fulfilling in this sense. What do they all have in common? They are all things that make you feel good about yourself, things that supply something you need.

If that is all that is meant by the claim that pregnancy is fulfilling, it strikes me as a reasonable description; but only so long as it is recognized that there is nothing necessary about this. That is, some women find pregnancy fulfilling and some do not. That idea is reasonable and certainly true; but it does not come close to capturing the sense of "fulfilling" used by, say, Helene Deutsch. Nor would it support the kind of intensely desperate reaction some women have at not experiencing pregnancy. Nor, to my mind, does it suggest that pregnancy is so significant as to justify a need for postmenopausal pregnancy in most cases.

So there is a stronger sense of "fulfilling" which may correspond more closely to the verb, "fulfill," meaning "to fill or accomplish." This is the sense assumed by gynecologists and psychologists, like Dirix, Deutsch, or Erikson, a sense that ascribes to all women a biological need to be pregnant, to fill their emptiness, to feel themselves as accomplishing womanhood by pregnancy.

It is this sense of fulfillment that imports a single mission to all women and implies the deficiency of all who do not meet it, or in some cases, who do not meet it often enough. It is this sense of fulfillment that assumes a single psychology for all women and suggests the maladjustment of those who diverge. And it is this complex of ideas that glorifies the experience of pregnancy in a way that most clearly supports the opportunity of postmenopausal pregnancy as a boon to women. But this idea of fulfillment is pernicious and false and needs to be abandoned. Thus, I must conclude that, like biological fatherhood, pregnancy may in most cases be a convenient means of obtaining a child, but it has no intrinsic value in and of itself.

Please do not misunderstand me. I am not saying that people ought not to have families. I am not saying that women ought not to have babies. And I am not saying that they ought not to be pleased about it. What I am suggesting is that we need to stop perpetuating myths of male immortality and female fulfillment that glorify pregnancy in a way that causes anguish and suffering among those who discover that it is not available to them, at least not without the heroic (and expensive) intervention of medical science. These myths encourage women to reject the natural aging process which affects one aspect of their lives but certainly not their basic identity as women or as human beings.

Think about it. In an overpopulated world, why is individual infertility a problem at all? It is only a problem because we have so greatly glorified biological parenthood, so tied it to self-esteem, so connected it to basic standards of adequacy for men and women for centuries, that those who cannot achieve it feel either unbearably deficient or tragically deprived. Either you are a failure as a woman or man, or you have been denied the gift of immortality and fulfillment. These attitudes were once pervasive. But that is no longer true, at least not universally true. The culture based on the significance of the seed and the glorification of pregnancy is disintegrating. It is much less uniformly effective than it once was; but it is still widely influential. What we should recognize and remember is that the freedom of women depends on its demise.

I am glad that medical science has provided new options for infertile women. (It has not cured infertility.) An infertile woman can now experience pregnancy by carrying an embryo from another woman. I hope that no woman feels compelled to accept this option as her only access to feminine fulfillment or her husband's immortality; but I fear that many who choose it will do so for exactly those reasons. I wish that we could (and I don't see why we can't) restructure our modern myths of male and female excellence, our standards of parenthood, and our procedures for adoption, so that no couple would think of resorting to this service until all homeless children have homes.

NOTES

1. For a trenchant first-hand description of this "cure," read *The Yellow Wallpaper* by Charlotte Perkins Gilman.

2. This, of course, was not a problem for the poor, as poor women were not educated in any case.

3. See also Barbre, "Meno-Boomers and Moral Guardians," in this volume, for further discussion of moral instruction in the guise of medical advice to women.

4. Recall that hysteria and depression were also diseases of the rich. Ovariotomies were not performed on the poor. In fact, it was widely held that the poor did not suffer from gynecological disorders, or even from general poor health. Fortunately, it has always been the rich, who can afford treatment, who tend to be sickly. As noted by D. Lucien Warner, "It is not then hard work and privation which make the women of our country invalids, but the so-called blessings of wealth and refinement" (109).

5. In "Egg Snatchers," Corea says, "Why are [men] splitting the functions of motherhood into smaller parts? Does that reduce the power of the mother and her claim to the child? ('I only gave the egg. I am not the real mother.' 'I only loaned the uterus. I am not the real mother.' 'I only raised the child. I am not the real mother.')"

6. But note that the only law we have yet on this matter has denied any rights at all to a gestational mother. The case of Baby Boy Johnson, decided 23 October 1990, in the California Superior Court, Orange County, cited in Pollitt. Perhaps Corea has a point.

7. Benedek says, for example, " . . . women incorporating the value-system of a modern society may develop personalities with rigid ego-defenses against their *biological needs*. The conflicts which arise from this can be observed clinically not only in the office of the psychiatrist, but also in the office of the gynecologist . . . " (emphasis added).

8. Interestingly, Deutsch would appear to have been a living counterexample to her own theory, unless she considered herself maladjusted. It is a fascinating question how conservative intellectual women manage to justify the contradiction between their own lives and their theories (see, e.g., Dworkin).

9. See Ehrenreich and English (chap. 8), for an impressive list.

10. If the contribution of writers to this cause is not obvious, just consider the subject matter of popular literature, movies, and TV programs of the 1950s and 1960s (such as "Father Knows Best," "Leave It to Beaver," or the whole series of Rock Hudson/Doris Day movies) or soap operas and romance novels even today.

11. It should be noted, however, that feminists laud the beneficial (or virtue-producing) qualities of motherhood as a whole. They do not ordinarily break it into pieces and discuss its separate parts. Nevertheless, some do rather glorify the special capacity women have to produce children.

12. Perhaps the real point is that figuring out how to take care of a baby at a basic level is not very hard. Any normal person could do it. It does not require special instinct, just common sense. The fact that women regularly figure out how to do it simply reflects the fact that they accept responsibility for the task. Nor does the fact that women themselves say things like "women just know these things" prove that women have special instinctive knowledge about child care. Women, like men, are conditioned to believe in mothers' instincts.

13. I am not claiming that there definitely are not human instincts. My claim rather consists of three points: (1) It is plausible to hold that human beings may have lost all, or virtually all instincts over time through the evolutionary process, and there is no way to tell at this point whether a trait is due to instinct or social conditioning. So claims about instincts are really assumptions; (2) It is also reasonable to think that if human beings do have any instincts, they do not have much intellectual content. Instincts are more like urges or feelings, such as "avoid death," or perhaps "protect your children." Instincts do not tell us how to do these things. Common sense or experience tell us that. Instincts (if we have them) do not inform; they motivate. So claiming that women (but not men) "just know" that babies get earaches if they go without hats, is silly; (3) If instincts are construed as basic, inarticulate urges to stay alive, or protect one's children, then there is no reason to attribute them to women but not to men. The existence of millions of very protective fathers is strong evidence against such a position.

REFERENCES

Barker-Benfield, G. J. 1976. *The Horrors of the Half-Known Life*. New York: Harper and Row.
Benedek, T., M.D. 1952. "Infertility as a Psychosomatic Disease." *Fertility and Sterility* 3:527.

Bullough, V. L., and Bullough, B. 1973. *The Subordinate Sex: A History of Attitudes toward Women.* Urbana: University of Illinois Press.
Clarke, E. H., M.D. 1972. *Sex in Education, Or a Fair Chance for the Girls* (1873). Reprinted, New York: Arno.
Corea, G. 1984. "Egg Snatchers." In *Test Tube Women: What Future for Motherhood?* Ed. R. Arditti, R. Klein, and S. Minden. London: Pandora. 45.
———. 1985. *The Mother Machine.* New York: Harper and Row.
Deutsch, H. 1944. *The Psychology of Women: A Psychoanalytic Interpretation.* Vol. 1. New York: Grune and Stratton.
Dirix, M. E., M.D. 1869. *Woman's Complete Guide to Health.* New York: Townsend and Adams.
Donchin, A. G. 1986. "The Future of Mothering: Reproductive Technology and Feminist Theory." *Hypatia* 1, no. 2 (Fall):131.
Dworkin, A. 1985. *Right-Wing Women.* New York: Dutton.
Ehrenreich, B., and English, D. 1978. *For Her Own Good.* New York: Doubleday.
Erikson, E. 1964. "The Inner and the Outer Space: Reflections on Womanhood." *Daedalus* 93, no. 2:582–606.
Firestone, S. 1970. *The Dialectic of Sex.* New York: Bantam.
Gilman, C. P. 1973. *The Yellow Wallpaper* (1899). Reprinted, New York: Feminist Press.
Goodman, E. 1990. "Doctors Discover a Way for Females to Beat Fertility Deadline." Syndicated column, *Springfield Union News,* 6 November. 11.
Hall, W. S., M.D. 1916. *Sexual Knowledge.* Philadelphia: Winfield.
Haller, J. S., and Haller, R. M. 1974. *The Physician and Sexuality in Victorian America.* Urbana: University of Illinois Press.
Love, S. M., M.D. 1990. *Dr. Susan Love's Breast Book.* New York: Addison Wesley.
O'Brien, M. 1981. *The Politics of Reproduction.* Boston: Routledge and Kegan Paul.
———. 1989. *Reproducing the World.* Boulder: Westview.
Osofsky, H. J., M.D. 1967. "Women's Reactions to Pelvic Examinations." *Obstetrics and Gynecology* 30:146.
Pollitt, K. 1990. "When Is a Mother Not a Mother?" *The Nation,* 31 December. 1ff.
Rich, A. 1979. *Of Woman Born.* New York: Norton.
Sturgis, S. H., and Menzer-Benaron, D. 1962. *The Gynecological Patient: A Psycho-Endocrine Study.* New York: Grune and Stratton.
von Hayek, F. 1960. *The Constitution of Liberty.* Chicago: University of Chicago Press.
Warner, D. L. 1874. *A Popular Treatise on the Functions and Diseases of Woman.* New York: Manhattan.

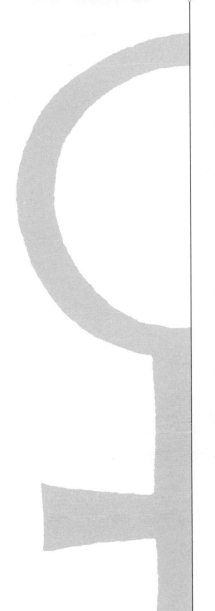

Part
Two

The Hormone
Replacement
Therapy
Debate

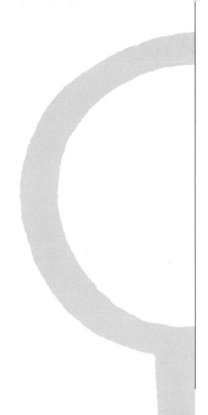

Disease or Development: Women's Perceptions of Menopause and the Need for Hormone Replacement Therapy

Mary Lou Logothetis

Menopause is a rite of passage for every woman who lives long enough. Given such a universal experience, one would think that a woman could count on clear guidelines and sound advice about what it means to her health. Yet differing perspectives on what menopause is and how it is best treated are hotly debated in the literature. Women are offered widely differing opinions and recommendations as to whether menopause is best defined as a disease or a developmental event and whether treatment and/or prevention of menopausal problems with hormone replacement therapy (HRT) is needed (Koninckx; MacPherson 1981, 1985; Utian 1987). When authorities present conflicting advice, a woman's ability to make an informed decision about HRT may be seriously compromised. My focus in this study is women's beliefs about menopause and their decision making regarding the use or nonuse of HRT.

The Medical Controversy

In order to appreciate the dilemma in which women find themselves with regard to differing advice about menopause and HRT, it is helpful to review the controversy depicted in the medical literature. Utian (1987) contended that the appropriate definition of menopause is at the forefront of current research. He noted that while some physicians define menopause as a natural event and regard attempts to correct decreasing hormone levels as meddlesome, other physicians define it as an endocrine dysfunction that needs correction with hormone replacement.

Brenner described the management of menopause as a medical dilemma of the twentieth century. Few other therapeutic regimens have generated as much debate as HRT. Some physicians believe HRT should be reserved for severe hot flashes and night sweats, vaginal dryness that leads to painful intercourse, or the prevention of osteoporosis in the small percent of women who are particularly susceptible (Cali; Edman; Judd et al.). The American Medical Association's Council on Scientific Affairs, the National Institutes of Health's Institute on Aging (Gastel et al.), and the World Health Organization all recommend a conservative use of HRT at the lowest possible dose for the shortest period of time.

A more liberal approach to HRT is recommended by other physicians who define menopause as a hormonal disease. These physicians advocate routine and long-term HRT, even in the absence of troubling symptoms, to prevent psychological problems, cardiovascular disease, and osteoporosis (Ettinger; Gambrell and Greenblatt; Hammond and Nachtigall). Drawing analogies between diabetes, a disease of insulin deficiency, and menopause, a disease of estrogen deficiency, Rauramo asserted that it is just as natural to give HRT to menopausal women as it is to give insulin to diabetic patients.

When women are exposed to such conflicting recommendations, the question of the impact on their ability to make informed decisions about HRT immediately arises. Specific investigations of women's beliefs and decisions about HRT, however, are sparse.

I used both quantitative and qualitative approaches to investigate what women themselves believe about menopause and the HRT controversy. In Section One, I report on quantitative data subjected to rigorous testing of a research hypothesis and analyzed through a structured format. In Section Two, I follow a more loosely structured format and use subjects' comments to describe menopausal experiences as lived and defined by the women themselves.

Section One

I selected the Health Belief Model (HBM) as the theoretical framework for the study, since this model has been found useful in understanding a variety of health-related behaviors. The HBM is based on the belief that the combined perception of four variables, susceptibility, seriousness, benefits, and barriers, determine an individual's health-related behavior (Rosenstock 1966, 1974). Thus, according to the model, women's perceptions regarding their susceptibility to menopausal problems, the seriousness of menopausal problems, and the benefits of HRT weighed against the barriers to HRT are expected to influence their decisions to use or not use the therapy. I added another variable, philosophical orientation to menopause, which measured women's perceptions about definitions of menopause, ranging from disease to development, in an attempt to enhance the HBM's ability to explain HRT use. I measured women's views on a continuum ranging from a disease to a developmental orientation to see if women, like physicians, disagree about whether menopause is normal physiology or a disease to be medically treated. My hypothesis tested for differences between users and nonusers of HRT for the variables of susceptibility, seriousness, benefits, barriers, and philosophical orientation to menopause.

The Sample

I recruited a convenience sample from a variety of women's organizations, such as women's clubs, social sororities, business and professional groups, and hospital volunteer groups, and distributed questionnaires at scheduled meetings. Responses from women in the climacteric age range of forty to sixty who had intact ovaries and were experiencing a natural menopause yielded a sample of 252. The subjects represented a homogeneous group of middle- to upper-class women who were highly educated; over 55% had completed college and almost one-fourth had completed graduate school.

The group included 36% premenopausal women (regular periods not more than three months apart), 9.5% perimenopausal women (irregular periods more than three months apart but not more than twelve months apart), 34.5% postmenopausal women (periods absent for more than twelve months), and 20% hysterectomized women (uterus removed with at least one ovary intact).

Symptom Experiences

Responses indicated that, overall, the women had not experienced high levels of menopausal distress.[1] To avoid bias, I gathered data about the nature of symptoms through open-ended questions rather than a symptom checklist.

Nearly 60% of the women attributed some type of symptom experience to menopause. The most commonly reported experience was the hot flash, mentioned by almost half of the women. Other experiences included weight gain and fluid retention, flooding and heavy periods, musculoskeletal pain, heart palpitations, and dizziness.

Although there is consensus in the medical literature that hot flashes and vaginal dryness are the only two phenomena directly attributable to the decreased hormone levels of menopause (Ballinger; Utian 1980), almost 20% of the women in this study reported an experience that included psychological problems. The women who attributed psychological experiences such as emotional lability, depression, anxiety, irritability, nervousness, and insomnia to their menopause also ranked their perceptions of distress higher than did those experiencing only physical changes.

Patterns of HRT Use

Almost 28% of the women were either currently using or had used HRT in the past. A total of 48% of women who reported both physical and psychological experiences also reported using HRT, while 35.4% of women reporting only physical experiences also reported using HRT. Postmenopausal women (41%) and hysterectomized women (39%) comprised the largest groups reporting past or current use. Only 11% of the perimenopausal women and 9% of the premenopausal women had ever used HRT.

Although long-term use of HRT is currently recommended by many physicians as a preventive health measure, use by these women was primarily short term and for symptom relief. Only 10% mentioned prevention of osteoporosis and/or heart disease when asked their reasons for using HRT, and almost 75% reported less than two years use. Whether the women were uninformed about or clearly rejected the notion of preventive use of HRT is uncertain.

I also asked women who were past users to share their reasons for discontinuing HRT. The most common response was a judgment that the therapy was no longer needed. Two other responses, fear of cancer and resumption of menstrual periods, are consistent with reports in the medical literature as to why women are reluctant to use HRT for long durations (Brenner; Ravnikar).

Findings and Discussion

I asked the women to respond to thirty-six items designed to measure the variables of susceptibility, seriousness, benefits, barriers, and philosophical orientation to menopause, by indicating their beliefs on a five-point scale that ranged from "strongly disagree" to "strongly agree." Representative items are presented in the table. The women, overall, did not feel highly susceptible to menopausal problems, did not perceive menopausal problems as serious, had stronger perceptions of the barriers to using HRT than of the benefits, and were undecided as to whether or not menopause is a medical event. Findings are consistent with studies using nonclinical groups of well women that have shown that, generally, although middle-aged women attribute some inconvenience to menopause, they do not regard it as a particularly threatening or serious event (Ballinger; McKinlay and Jefferys; Neugarten et al.). That women, even as highly educated as those in this sample, should express uncertainty as to whether menopause is a medical event is not surprising and may well be a reflection of the lack of agreement within the medical profession about the long-term consequences of menopause.

I found that current users of HRT had significantly stronger perceptions of susceptibility to and seriousness of menopausal problems, of HRT's benefits, and of menopause as a medical event than did nonusers.[2] The variable most successful at accounting for differences was the benefits/barriers variable, while the second most successful variable was the philosophical orientation to menopause.

The decisions made by the women in this study were based mainly on their perceptions of HRT's benefits weighed against its barriers and their orientations to menopause as disease or development. Perceptions of how susceptible the women felt to menopausal problems in the future or how seriously they regarded the consequences of menopause did not play a major role in their decisions about HRT, a finding clearly in contrast to current medical recommendations, which point to menopause as a significant factor in later-life health problems, such as osteoporosis and cardiovascular disease.

Section Two

While the study's findings shed light on women's beliefs about menopause and HRT, they fall short of communicating the inherent richness and complexity of their thoughts. The purpose of this section is to complement the quantitative data reported in Section One and lend insight into the meanings women attach to their lived experiences of menopause.

At the end of the questionnaire, I included an invitation to the women to elaborate on their thoughts about menopause and HRT. Several recur-

TABLE: Representative Items on Questionnaire

Susceptibility
I don't believe I will have trouble with menopause.
My health status makes having problems with menopause likely.

Seriousness
Menopausal problems may threaten my health.
Problems associated with going through menopause are small.

Benefits
Taking estrogen can help me maintain my health.
I have a lot to gain by taking estrogen.

Barriers
Side effects from estrogen can be harmful to my health.
The disadvantages of estrogen therapy outweigh any advantages.

Philosophical Orientation to Menopause
A woman should consult her physician as soon as she suspects she is in menopause.
Menopause can be a time of personal growth for women.

rent patterns and themes emerged in the responses. Even the degree of response to the invitation was revealing. Of the 252 subjects, only a handful chose not to respond. Most filled the entire page provided; many took even more space. Obviously, women want to talk about this subject and they have much to say.

The meanings attached to menopause by the women of this sample were overwhelmingly positive. A frequently expressed theme depicted menopause as a challenge and an opportunity for further female development. Representative comments included "a period of reflection, to reassess life's goals," "a new beginning," and "change, growth, and new directions."

Most women placed menopause within an overall context of their menstrual and reproductive lives. The majority of women linked menopause to the end of menstruation and considered it a relief from what they seemed to regard as a monthly nuisance. Many conveyed a sense of fortitude in controlling any discomforts, saying, for example, "It's like your period—it's what you make of it, good or bad," and "I just don't let menopause get to me." Others attached less inconvenience to menopause than to their earlier menstrual years, with comments such as "I had more discomfort from periods than from menopause," and "If I can tolerate PMS, I can tolerate menopause." Many of the women depicted menopause as a marker of the end of childbearing; however, they did so, not within a context of regret or loss, but one of appreciation and anticipation for a new, nonfertile state. A common statement was "No more fear of getting pregnant." There was no expression of the so-called "empty nest syndrome" in this sample. Rather, the women frequently communicated a sense of freedom from the responsibility of bearing and nurturing children. The women's responses support earlier evidence that healthy women express relief rather than regret over the cessation of their periods, and that loss of reproductive capacity is not an important concern to midlife women (Neugarten et al.; McKinlay and Jefferys; Severne).

The positive pattern in these women's responses may reflect the relatively high socioeconomic and educational levels of the sample. Other studies have also demonstrated the tendency of upper-class and highly educated women to express more positive views of menopause (Dege and Gretzinger; Severne). Less than 10% of the women expressed pessimistic attitudes that equated menopause with symptoms of distress and ill health, such as "An upheaval in my life," and "It's a sickness and should be treated as such."

While the meanings these women attached to menopause were somewhat homogeneous, their perceptions about HRT are not so easily summarized. Indeed, their perspectives seem as varied as those of the professionals currently engaged in debate.

Women who had never used HRT questioned its value. One asked, "Why cause a bigger problem than the one you're trying to cure?" and another asserted, "Leaning on estrogen or other medications seems like trying to blot out an uncomfortable but quite natural process." A forty-eight-year-old woman said, "I have a bottle on my shelf prescribed last spring. Too busy with all the good things in my life and forgot to take it. I'm not really sure it will make much difference in me." A fifty-nine-year-old postmenopausal woman, pleased that she had "survived hot flashes without medication, and did not seek medical attention as I didn't feel it necessary," at the same time wondered, "Is something wrong with me?"

Even current users expressed reservations and concerns about the effects of HRT. One woman, for example, remarked that after two months of using HRT, "I am concerned with the effect this will have on me, although I seem to feel better." A forty-seven-year-old user commented, "I have very mixed feelings about using estrogen. I gave up using birth control pills nineteen years ago because I was afraid of side effects, and am still faced with the same kind of fears." Another woman expressed her fears more specifically when she said, "There has got to be a better HRT program for women. I've had breast surgery after my initial estrogen therapy. I've now started again. Since my mother died of breast cancer, I worry about it a great deal."

The concern with HRT's relationship to breast cancer was raised by others, creating a distinct pattern in the responses. Many women explained that they do not define themselves as candidates for HRT because they have a family history of breast cancer or because they have had either benign or malignant breast tumors. One example was a fifty-one-year-old postmenopausal woman who explained, "My medical and genetic background make me an above average risk for breast cancer and osteoporosis. I've conferred with my doctor and my gynecologist. My choice is to avoid estrogen. I prefer to take my chances with osteoporosis over taking chances with breast cancer, questions which for me haven't been resolved by medical science."

These reservations about HRT contrast with the comments from users and past users who were firmly convinced of its value. Two women rejoiced, "Thank God I live in an era of medical assistance for easing the symptoms of discomfort . . . menopause can be a time of growth and productivity" (after two years use), and "I know I have felt miserable and couldn't figure out why. . . . It's an expense not everyone could afford, but thank God I can" (after five years use). A postmenopausal past user who had used HRT for eight years, then stopped because she felt she did not need it any longer, was adamant, "If I had to go through it again, I'd take estrogen." After four months of use, another woman said, "I went through menopause for five years before I went to my doctor for help. The hot flashes were embarrassing in public and the depression I was going through was not me. I trust my doctor and I feel that taking the estrogen has helped me." A seven-year user of the therapy exclaimed, "I tried not taking Premarin—it was awful!!"

Two other current HRT users (each for two years) pointed out significant menopausal effects on their health and well-being which they were certain had been relieved by the therapy. The first woman had suffered pain in joints, bones, jaws, along with severe exhaustion, and said, "When estrogen was prescribed, the overall pain relief was astounding, and for the first time, I connected the problems to the cause. I still experience aching during the five days each month my physician requires me to go off estrogen, and I wish I never had to, but he feels it is a safer way to take it." The second woman exclaimed, "I am bitter that I lost two teeth and three-fourths inches in height before my doctor, whom I saw yearly for check-ups, prescribed estrogen."

This woman's bitterness leads to another recurrent theme that emerged from the data. Many of the women expressed a strong sense of dissatisfaction with their physicians and the advice they had been offered. One woman was grateful that her severe distress was greatly improved with HRT, but she complained that to get it prescribed, she had to "finally scream" at her doctor that she "needed estrogen." Another woman told a similar story, saying "I had to insist that my OB/Gyn place me on hormonal therapy." She described her physician as conservative, but said she did not want to leave him because she felt she could "perhaps educate him on menopause." She concluded that, after four years of HRT use, "it has worked out well."

Other subjects judged their physicians as less than knowledgeable about menopause and unconcerned with educating women about what to expect in the transition. As one woman said, "I feel the best qualified physicians know less about menopause than any other part of medicine. When they disagree on HRT it causes me to be less inclined to use it." Another charged that "there are far too many paternal physicians in this world who would rather turn to the prescription pad than take the time to educate their patients." Still another questioned in frustration, "My male physician offers very little information or help concerning menopause. I have gone to him for twenty-five years and hate to change. What can be done to give these men more tools to handle this stage in life?" There seemed to be a sense among many of the women that female physicians would be more sympathetic, best expressed by this fifty-eight-year-old's comment, "Men do not know how a woman feels and experiences maternity and the years following, as well as menopause. I hope more women become OB/Gyn specialists, have intercourse, conceive, deliver, and then experience menopause . . . then I'll believe the physicians who say 'they know.' "

Three final themes emerged which deserve mention. The first is skepticism, represented by the comments of a forty-five-year-old woman who linked HRT with profit motives and suggested there be no more drug development until more is known about the menopausal process. She said, "I am concerned about research of menopausal problems. The research done by pharmaceutical companies will not be toward the benefit of females, only the benefit of the company. Support for research on the normal and the problematic must come from neutral areas."

Responses from two HRT users are examples of an additional theme of ambivalence. One woman raved about how much better she felt after starting HRT, but then added, "The thought of taking estrogen the rest of my life is depressing." The other noted, "I already feel better" (after four months use), but then added, "I'm still not completely convinced if it's safe." Comments from a forty-eight-year-old premenopausal woman who had never used HRT also revealed ambivalence. She warned, "We need to be careful about HRT. I don't believe there's a pill to cure everything, nor do I believe all our discomforts can be alleviated." Yet she left the door open to the possibility of a different view, saying, "I may, of course, change my mind if and when it hits me hard!"

The final theme was one of yearning. Many women yearned for HRT's benefits, represented by one woman with a history of breast cancer who stated, "I wish I could take it; it may help my libido. I've not had an orgasm for two years." Another woman, who first described how she had discontinued HRT use after six months because her breasts swelled and ached so that she could no longer stand it, then added, "but I felt so wonderful otherwise." Other women yearned for different choices, summarized by the comment, "I wish there were other options than estrogen. We all just assume estrogen and menopause go hand-in-hand." Still other women yearned for answers about risks and benefits. A fifty-one-year-old nonuser pondered, "I am concerned with its unknown effects. I'm strongly considering it and wish I knew the correct answer," while another woman remarked, "I wish I knew the answer. . . . I truly wish I knew if HRT is safe!" Finally, one woman referred to what she perceived as a multitude of conflicting opinions about HRT and said, "I wish there were more discussion of this in the media and more research done so we women could make more informed decisions."

Conclusion

The results of my study suggest that the most important variable in a woman's decision making about HRT is her perception of its benefits weighed against its barriers. Since there is currently no uniform recommendation applicable to all women as to whether HRT should or should not be used, each woman must make the decision for herself. In order to make an intelligent choice, she needs as much information as possible about the benefits and risks in general, as well as those applicable to her unique situation. The comments of many women in this sample make it clear that women perceive a need for more understandable and reliable information about menopause and HRT in order to make an informed choice about HRT.

Although health care professionals can and should use every opportunity to teach women about HRT, a large portion of the educational burden will continue to fall on individual women. As long as HRT remains at all controversial, every woman will need to make every effort to understand the potential benefits and the potential risks of HRT rather than passively accepting whatever others tell her. Health care professionals, in turn, must respect women's freedom of choice and do their best to provide complete and unbiased education on menopause and HRT, thereby facilitating decisions by their clients. Warner stressed that consent cannot be free unless the person is in "the best possible position to weigh the risks against [her] own individual subjective fears and hopes" (27). Health care professionals need to regard their charge as experts as putting their clients in this best possible position by disclosing to them the available relevant data and then standing back. Such a posture leaves women free to make what are more than purely medical judgments, since they involve an understanding of each woman's individual priorities, beliefs, and concerns—an understanding that is not fully accessible to a health-care professional.

NOTES

1. I asked the women to indicate on a scale of 0–10 the highest level of menopausal distress they had ever experienced. The mean response was 2.8. Nearly 75% of the women indicated no distress or distress at a minimal level below 4. Only 7% rated their distress as severe at levels of 8–10 on the scale.

2. I tested the hypothesis that users and nonusers of HRT would have significantly different beliefs for the variables of susceptibility, seriousness, benefits, barriers, and philosophical orientation to menopause with a MANCOVA analysis that controlled for the extraneous variable of perceived menopausal distress ($p < .000$). Complete detail on statistical procedures and results can be found in my article "Women's decisions about estrogen replacement therapy" (*Western Journal of Nursing Research* 13, no. 4[1991]:458–74).

REFERENCES

Ballinger, S. 1985. Psychosocial stress and symptoms of menopause: A comparative study of menopause clinic patients and nonpatients. *Maturitas* 7:315–27.

Brenner, P. 1982. The menopause. *The Western Journal of Medicine* 136 (3):211–19.

Cali, R. 1984. Estrogen replacement therapy—boon or bane? *Postgraduate Medicine* 75 (4):279–86.

Council on Scientific Affairs, American Medical Association. 1983. Estrogen replacement in the menopause. *Journal of the American Medical Association* 249 (3):359–61.

Dege, K., and J. Gretzinger. 1982. Attitudes of families toward menopause. In A. Voda, M. Dinnerstein, and S. O'Donnell, eds., *Changing perspectives on menopause*. Austin: University of Texas Press. 60–69.

Edman, C. 1983. Estrogen replacement therapy. In H. Buchsbaum, ed., *The menopause*. New York: Springer-Verlag. 77–83.

Ettinger, B. 1987. Overview of the efficacy of hormonal replacement therapy. *American Journal of Obstetrics and Gynecology* 156:1298–1303.

Gambrell, R., and R. Greenblatt. 1981. Hormone therapy for the menopause. *Geriatrics* 36 (7):53–61.

Gastel, B., J. Cornoni-Hunley, and J. Brody. 1980. Estrogen use and postmenopausal women: A basis for informed decisions. *Journal of Family Practice* 11 (6):851–60.

Hammond, C., and L. Nachtigall. 1985. Is estrogen therapy necessary? *Journal of Reproductive Medicine* 30 (10):797–800.

Judd, H., R. Cleary, W. Creasman, D. Figge, N. Kase, Z. Rosenwaks, and G. Tagatz. 1981. Estrogen replacement therapy. *Obstetrics and Gynecology* 58 (3):267–75.

Koninckx, P. 1983. Menopause: The beginning of a curable disease or a lucky phenomenon? In H. van Herendael, R. Riphagen, L. Goessens, and H. van der Pas, eds., *The climacteric: Proceedings of the 4th European conference on menopause*. Boston: MTP Press. 3–18.

MacPherson, K. 1981. Menopause as disease: The social construction of a metaphor. *Advances in Nursing Science* 3 (2):95–113.

———. 1985. Osteoporosis and menopause: A feminist analysis of the social construction of a syndrome. *Advances in Nursing Science* 7 (4):11–22.

McKinlay, S., and M. Jefferys. 1974. The menopausal syndrome. *British Journal of Preventive and Social Medicine* 28:108–15.

Neugarten, B., V. Wood, R. Kraines, and B. Loomis. 1963. Women's attitudes toward the menopause. *Vita Humana* 6 (3):140–51.

Rauramo, L. 1986. A review of study findings of the risks and benefits of estrogen therapy in the female climacteric. *Maturitas* 8:177 86.

Ravnikar, V. 1987. Compliance with hormone therapy. *American Journal of Obstetrics and Gynecology* 156:1332–34.

Rosenstock, I. 1966. Why people use health services. *Milbank Memorial Fund Quarterly* 44:94–127.

———. 1974. Historical origins of the health belief model. In M. Becker, ed., *The health belief model and personal health behavior*. Thorofare, N.J.: Charles B. Slack. 1–8.

Severne, L. 1979. Psycho-social aspects of the menopause. In A. Haspels and H. Musaph, eds., *Psychosomatics in peri-menopause*. Lancaster: MTP Press.

Utian, W. 1980. *Menopause in modern perspective*. New York: Appleton-Century-Crofts.

———. 1987. Overview on menopause. *American Journal of Obstetrics and Gynecology* 156:1280–83.

Warner, R. 1980. *Morality in medicine: An introduction to medical ethics.* Sherman Oaks, Calif.: Alfred.

World Health Organization. 1982. Research on the menopause. *The Lancet* 2:137–38.

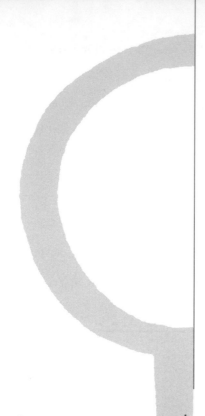

Making a Reasoned Choice about Hormone Replacement Therapy

Susan R. Johnson and
Kristi J. Ferguson

As women live longer, their number of years after menopause continues to increase. Currently, most women can expect to spend twenty-five to thirty years, or about one-third of their lives, after menopause. Because the disorders that are associated with estrogen deficiency are among the major causes of morbidity and mortality in this age group, every woman should understand the issues surrounding hormone replacement therapy.

The decision to use hormone replacement therapy (HRT) should be a mutual one between an individual woman and her physician. In order to make a reasoned choice about HRT, women who are medically eligible should carefully weigh the costs and benefits not only of the treatment, but of the alternatives, including that of no treatment. The final decision should be based on what is important to each individual woman. This paper will outline what is currently known (and not known) about these potential risks and benefits and then will summarize a study done by the authors on women's knowledge and attitudes about HRT, which suggests that many women are not well informed about hormone replacement therapy.

It is useful to conceptualize HRT as being given either over a relatively short period of time for the relief of acute estrogen deficiency symptoms (e.g., hot flushes or flashes), or indefinitely for the prevention of certain systemic changes related to loss of estrogen (e.g., osteoporosis). It is the latter use that generates most of the controversy; consequently this paper will focus primarily on hormones given for the purpose of "prophylaxis."

Short-Term HRT Use

There are few risks, and much symptomatic relief to be gained, with short-term estrogen administration for treatment of menopausal symptoms (Mishell; Notelovitz). These symptoms include hot flashes, sweating, sleep problems, vaginal dryness and thinning of the vaginal walls, and painful intercourse. Although none of these symptoms is life-threatening, and some will eventually go away on their own, any of these can produce considerable discomfort.

Hot flashes provide a good example. For some women, they are merely an inconvenience, to be tolerated and perhaps joked about, but not severe enough to require hormone therapy. For others, night-time hot flashes result in waking up, as often as every fifteen minutes. The resultant sleep disruption can lead to psychological problems such as depression, irritability, and difficulty with cognitive functioning. Hormone therapy, taken from several months up to a few years, is the most effective treatment for this problem.

Other common problems are vaginal dryness and thinning of the vaginal walls which can interfere with intercourse. Some have suggested that water soluble lubricants, such as KY jelly, are preferable to estrogen creams. While lubricants may be sufficient for women who have regular vaginal intercourse throughout menopause, women who do not have regular intercourse or who stop for a while and wish to start again may need estrogen creams to restore vaginal function.

Long-Term HRT Use

One of the long-term changes associated with estrogen deficiency is osteoporosis. Although estimates of the age at which women reach their peak bone mass vary, most agree that by age thirty-five women begin to lose bone mass. Being a woman and being white both place one at increased risk of osteoporosis. Dietary calcium and weight-bearing exercise, or exercise that involves putting weight on bones and joints, can reduce risk of osteoporosis. All of these factors influence how much bone mass a woman has when the process of losing bone mass begins. Even women who have substantial bone mass as they approach menopause will lose fifteen percent of their bone mass every ten years after menopause if they do not take hormone replacement therapy. This bone loss can have very serious consequences.

For example, osteoporosis is an important factor in eighty percent of the 120,000 hip fractures in elderly women each year. Statistics suggest that one out of every six individuals with a hip fracture will die within three months of sustaining the fracture. Even when death does not occur, fractures can lead to prolonged loss of mobility; many otherwise healthy elderly women must give up independent living after a hip fracture. Twenty-five percent of women over age sixty, and eighty percent of women over age seventy-five have spinal compression fractures leading not only to loss of weight, but to chronic pain and occasionally significant respiratory problems because of interference in the normal mechanisms of breathing.

Obviously, not all menopausal women sustain bone fractures, so that universal HRT should not be recommended simply for this purpose. It would be helpful if it were possible to identify women at high risk for osteoporosis-related fractures, so that HRT could be prescribed more selectively. The known risk factors for osteoporosis (sex, age, race, family history, weight, smoking, urinary calcium excretion) are suggestive, but not selective enough. There is considerable interest in using the measurement of bone mineral density as a selection criterion. Basically, this test measures how thick (or thin) the bone is. It is known that postmenopausal women who have bone thickness in the lowest twenty-five percent have three times the risk of fracture as those with normal bone thickness. This test, therefore, may help some women to decide about taking HRT. It is important to remember, however, that women outside of this high-risk range of bone thickness also continue to lose bone in menopause and do have a real, although smaller, risk of fractures. Further, routine testing for bone mineral density is not yet recommended, since its cost-effectiveness has not yet been tested (Melton, et al.).

Several options for reducing the rate of bone loss have been suggested as alternatives to HRT. For example, increasing dietary and other sources of calcium has been promoted heavily in recent years. Unfortunately, postponing calcium supplements until after menopause has occurred may not slow down bone loss enough to reduce fracture rates; new evidence suggests that calcium intake must be increased as early as the third decade of life for it to be effective. Other dietary supplements such as fluoride and vitamin D, while important elements in normal bone metabolism, also do not provide a significant effect, either alone or in combination. Regular, weight-bearing exercise also helps build up bone mass in the years before menopause and may help slow down the rate of bone loss after menopause. But neither dietary supplements (including calcium) nor weight-bearing exercise is as effective at preventing osteoporosis as HRT, which a

National Institutes of Health consensus conference determined was the most effective single modality for the prevention of osteoporosis in women (Ettinger).

Finally, some have suggested that preventing falls may be a safer and more direct way to reduce the serious fractures associated with osteoporosis. Unfortunately, many of the events that lead to fractures may be relatively ordinary activities, for example, lifting a basket of laundry or opening a door, and some compression fractures may occur with no trauma at all, for example, when an individual is standing or walking.

In sum, there is now a wealth of medical evidence that HRT can control the symptoms of menopause for those women who have problems, and that long-term administration of estrogen can reduce both the development of osteoporosis and the rate of serious fractures.

Current interest is focused on the effect of HRT on risk of heart disease. Heart disease (and in particular heart attack) is the leading cause of death in postmenopausal women, far outweighing death caused by cancer or fractures (Hazzard). There is substantial epidemiologic evidence suggesting that HRT with estrogen alone reduces deaths in postmenopausal women that are related to heart disease (Bush, et al.).

For example, in women aged forty-five to forty-nine, the number of heart attacks per year is 2 per 1,000 in women who have not gone through menopause and 4 per 1,000 in women who have. Among women aged fifty to fifty-four, the numbers are 3.6 for women who have not gone through menopause and 6.5 for those who have. In each group, postmenopausal women have two to five times as many heart attacks as premenopausal women. Looked at another way, as many menopausal women over fifty die of heart attacks as men of the same age. Although the exact reason for the statistical relationship between menopausal status and increased heart disease risk has not been firmly established, it is known that loss of estrogen increases LDL, the so-called bad cholesterol, and decreases HDL, the so-called good cholesterol, resulting in an increased risk profile (Matthews et al.). There are retrospective studies that show that women using estrogen have half the number of heart attacks of those who do not. It is important to realize that if this preventive role of estrogen is real, the number of lives saved using estrogen for this reason alone may outweigh any of the known or hypothesized risks of HRT.

There are potential problems, however, associated with giving estrogen alone to women with a uterus. Because estrogen stimulates the lining of the uterus, a small number of women will develop a condition called "endometrial hyperplasia," which can be precancerous, and if proper treatment is not given, a small number of women will develop endometrial cancer (Henderson). Women who take estrogen in menopause have about twice the risk of endometrial cancer as women who do not. The actual number of cancers is quite low: about 3 per 1000 women not on estrogen, and 6 per 1000 who take it. The risk goes up the longer the estrogen is used, and it may reach an eight-fold risk after more than eight years of use. The endometrial cancer that develops as a result of estrogen exposure can usually be treated with a hysterectomy, and the overall cure rate is in excess of ninety-five percent. In fact, there is evidence that, overall, women who develop this kind of cancer do not have any shortening of their life spans. We do not want to suggest that getting endometrial cancer is a trivial matter. It certainly is not. Major surgery is required for therapy, and a few women will have more advanced disease that cannot be cured as easily. Nonetheless, relative to the problems of osteoporosis and heart disease, both the actual occurrence rate and the mortality rate of endometrial cancer are quite low.

With regular checkups, women at risk for endometrial cancer can usually have this problem discovered in the precancerous (hyperplasia) stage and can be treated with simple medical therapy. In addition, both hyperplasia and endometrial cancer can be prevented by giving a progesterone-type hormone (or "progestin") along with the estrogen. For this reason, the most common current practice is to prescribe progestin along with estrogen for women who still have a uterus (DeFazio and Speroff).

Unfortunately, the use of progestin raises an additional question that has not yet been answered: How does adding progestins affect the risk of heart disease? Theoretically, progestins may neutralize, or even reverse, the cardiovascular benefits of estrogen related to cholesterol. Studies done in the past are reassuring insofar as they show that the most commonly used progestin in the United States, medroxyprogesterone acetate, has relatively weak lipid effects and so may not counteract the effects of the estrogen. Two recently published studies showed that women taking combination estrogen/progestin therapy had the same beneficial changes in cholesterol levels as women who were taking estrogen by itself (Barrett-Conner, et al.; Egeland, et al.).

This issue requires further investigation, however. In addition to determining more about the effects of the progestins currently in use, there are newer types of progestin being studied that may not have any adverse lipid effects. The study, called the Postmenopausal Estrogen Progestin Intervention trial (PEPI), has randomly assigned approximately nine hundred women for three years each to either estrogen alone, placebo, or one of three estrogen/progestin combinations. The researchers will compare the effects of the different treatments on several heart disease risk factors, including cholesterol. Among other things, PEPI is also assessing effects of the hormones on quality of life issues, including medication side effects, bleeding patterns, and sexual functioning.

What about other potential risks of HRT? In some lay (and even medical) literature about HRT, the impression is given that menopausal HRT and oral contraceptives are the same and are therefore associated with the same types of adverse effects. In fact, the hormones used in these two interventions are quite different, and, in particular, there is no association between HRT and thromboembolic disease (blood clots), stroke, high blood pressure, diabetes, or heart attack. Indeed, as we have already noted, HRT may actually prevent heart attacks.

Another concern that has been raised regarding HRT is its possible association with increased risk of breast cancer (Wingo et al.). A recent Swedish study showed an increased risk of breast cancer in a small group of women (Bergkvist et al.). Even though methodologic problems have been identified with that study, and other studies have not documented such a relationship (Barrett-Connor), the effect of HRT on risk for breast cancer needs continued study (Hammond). Even considering the results of the Bergkvist study, however, the overall maximum hypothesized increased risk is roughly no more than about 1.5 and appears to increase to this level only after prolonged use, that is, use in excess of ten years (Hulka).

This level of increased risk probably applies to women who are at average risk for breast cancer. Women who are at high risk (for example, with a first-degree relative such as a mother or sister who had premenopausal breast cancer) may increase their risk of breast cancer even more with many years of estrogen use. These women, therefore, will need to take this factor into account when weighing their individual overall potential benefits and risks. For example, if a woman at high risk of breast cancer has no risk factors (other than being postmenopausal) for heart disease and osteoporosis, she may very well conclude that the risks of HRT for her are greater than the potential benefits.

Finally, women with certain medical problems should not take HRT. These problems include previously diagnosed tumors that may be stimulated to grow by estrogen, such as in breast cancer, advanced endometrial (uterine) cancer, or malignant melanoma; currently active liver disease; and possible previous hormone-associated thromboembolic disease, although the evidence for this contraindication is weak.

Since most women do not have medical conditions that prohibit HRT, and there may be substantial benefit that, at least theoretically, far outweighs any risks, why is it so infrequently used? We recently conducted a survey of menopausal women to try to learn more about the answer to this question (Ferguson et al.). In addition to assessing the respondents' personal experience with HRT, we asked about their knowledge of osteoporosis, estrogen risks and benefits, attitudes toward menopause, and factors that would influence their own decision about HRT. In addition, we were particularly interested in determining the impact on these decisions of certain practical aspects of using HRT, such as the need to take drugs over a long period of time, the prospect of either regular monthly bleeding or unpredictable bleeding, and the extra testing necessary to monitor HRT (Hahn).

The groups included 37 women who were currently taking HRT and 125 other menopausal women who had never taken HRT. The survey found several significant knowledge gaps. For example, while nearly all of the women who were taking HRT knew that lack of estrogen was a risk factor in osteoporosis (eighty-nine percent correct), fewer than one-third of those who were not on HRT (twenty-seven percent) were aware of this association. Similarly, while nearly all of the women who were taking HRT knew that HRT could reduce the risk of osteoporosis (eighty-six percent correct), fewer than one-third of those not taking it (twenty-eight percent) were aware of this. Women in the study also differed regarding factors that influenced (or would influence) their decision to take HRT. Those currently on HRT said that its potential to stop hot flashes was a significant positive factor in their decisions, while its potential to cause periods was a significant negative factor. Women currently on HRT were also more likely than those not taking it to perceive menopause as a medical condition, to believe that women with distressing symptoms should be on HRT, and to see natural approaches to menopause as less preferable than taking hormones.

Contrary to reports that physicians universally (and by implication, indiscriminately) prescribe HRT (Eagan), this study found that most women who were potentially eligible (77/125 or sixty-two percent) had not even discussed the possibility of this treatment with their physicians. This is consistent with national survey data suggesting that only ten to fifteen percent of menopausal women are currently using HRT, with only five percent using it for at least ten years (Melton, et al.). In our survey, the most important factor a woman considered in making a decision about HRT was the advice of her physician.

In sum, there are many factors to consider in making an informed choice about hormone replacement therapy, and we do not recommend universal use of these drugs. The most important step in the decision-making process is to obtain accurate, balanced information about the potential health effects, both risks *and* benefits, associated with HRT. To summarize briefly, for women at higher than average risk of osteoporosis or heart disease, there is growing evidence that HRT will substantially reduce mortality from these conditions. On the other hand, women at high risk of breast cancer may want to avoid *long-term* use of estrogen. For women at average risk of these conditions, the benefits are of lower magnitude but are still significant, at least in terms of mortality rates. We believe that most women do not yet take the step of gathering this information, and we recommend that both women and their physicians actively address the question of HRT when menopause approaches.

REFERENCES

Barrett-Connor, E. 1989. Postmenopausal estrogen replacement and breast cancer. N. Engl. J. of Med. 321:319–20.

Barrett-Connor, E.; Wingard, D. L.; and Criqui, M. H. 1989. Postmenopausal estrogen use and heart disease risk factors in the 1980's: Rancho Bernardo, California, revisited. JAMA 261:2095–100.

Bergkvist, L.; Hans Olov, A.; Persson, I.; et al. 1989. The risk of breast cancer after estrogen and estrogen-progestin replacement. N. Engl. J. of Med. 321:293–97.

Bush, T. L.; Cowan, L. D.; Barrett-Connor, E.; et al. 1983. Estrogen use and all-cause mortality: Preliminary results from the Lipid Research Clinics Program Follow-Up Study. JAMA 249:903–906.

DeFazio, J., and Speroff, L. 1985. Estrogen replacement therapy: Current thinking and practice. Geriatrics 40:32–48.

Eagan, A. B. 1989. The estrogen fix. Ms. (April) 38–43.

Egeland, G. M.; Kuller, L. H.; Matthews, K. A.; Kelsey, S. F.; Cauley, J.; and Guzick, D. 1990. Hormone replacement therapy and lipoprotein changes during early menopause. Obstet. Gynecol. 76:776–82.

Elstein, A. S.; Holzman, G. B.; Ravitch, M. M.; et al. 1986. Comparison of physicians' decisions regarding estrogen replacement therapy for menopausal women and decisions derived from a decision analytic model. Am. J. of Med. 80:246–58.

Ettinger, B. 1987. Update: Estrogen and postmenopausal osteoporosis 1976–1986. Health Values 11:31–36.

Ferguson, K. J.; Hoegh, C.; and Johnson, S. 1989. Estrogen replacement therapy: A survey of women's knowledge and attitudes. Arch. of Int. Med. 149:133–36.

Genant, H. K.; Baylink, D. J.; and Gallagher, J. C. 1989. Estrogens in the prevention of osteoporosis in postmenopausal women. Amer. J. of Ob. and Gyn. 161:1842–46.

Hahn, R. G. 1989. Compliance considerations with estrogen replacement: Withdrawal bleeding and other factors. Amer. J. of Ob. and Gyn. 161:1854–58.

Hammond, C. B. 1989. Estrogen replacement therapy: What the future holds. Amer. J. of Ob. and Gyn. 161:1864–68.

Hazzard, W. R. 1989. Estrogen replacement and cardiovascular disease: Serum lipids and blood pressure effects. Am. J. of Ob. and Gyn. 161:1847–53.

Henderson, B. E. 1989. The cancer question: An overview of recent epidemiologic and retrospective data. Am. J. of Ob. and Gyn. 161:1859–63.

Holzman, G. B.; Ravitch, M. M.; Metheny, W.; et al. 1984. Physicians' judgments about estrogen replacement therapy for menopausal women. Ob. and Gyn. 63:303–11.

Hulka, B. S. 1990. Hormone-replacement therapy and the risk of breast cancer. CA—A Cancer Journal for Clinicians 40 (5):289–96.

Matthews, K. A.; Meilahn, E.; Kuller, L. H.; et al. 1989. Menopause and risk factors for coronary heart disease. N. Engl. J. of Med. 321:641–46.

Melton, L. J., 3d; Eddy, D. M.; and Johnston, C. C., Jr. 1990. Screening for osteoporosis. Ann. Intern. Med. 112:516–28.

Mishell, D. R. 1989. Estrogen replacement therapy: An overview. Am. J. of Ob. and Gyn. 161:1825–27.

Notelovitz, M. 1989. Estrogen replacement therapy: Indications, contraindications, and agent selection. Am. J. of Ob. and Gyn. 161:1832–41.

Ross, R. K.; Paganini-Hill, A.; Roy, S.; et al. 1988. Past and present preferred prescribing practices of hormone replacement therapy among Los Angeles gynecologists: Possible implications for public health. Am. J. of Pub. Health 78:516–19.

Wingo, P. A.; Layde, P. M.; Lee, N. C.; et al. 1987. The risk of breast cancer in postmenopausal women who have used estrogen replacement therapy. JAMA 257:209–15.

The False Promises of Hormone Replacement Therapy and Current Dilemmas

Kathleen I. MacPherson

In spite of the promises . . . estrogen is not the fountain of youth. No drug has been found which stops or turns back the normal aging process.

—*Montreal Health Press*

Menopause has been medicalized (Zola) by calling it a disease or a syndrome that requires hormonal intervention. Feminist scholars, health activists, and many other women have learned to question the objectivity and neutrality of patriarchal science, particularly in regard to scientific ideas generated about women's bodies (Hubbard and Lowe).

Medicine uses science to legitimate the power of physicians to define both illness and its treatment. Yet evidence abounds, as in the case of widespread prescriptions of diethylstilbestrol (DES) to prevent spontaneous abortion and premature labor, that the claim of therapeutic gain has sometimes been used to justify medical intervention even when the scientific evidence was unconfirmed or contradictory (Bell). Feminist distrust (Reinharz) is called for when examining much of the medical menopausal research and most certainly the motives of transnational pharmaceutical companies that manufacture hormones.

Three kinds of false promises have been made to women by biomedical researchers, physicians, mass media, and pharmaceutical companies about the benefits of hormone treatments. These promises can best be examined chronologically to facilitate an understanding of how the rationales for prescribing hormones for menopause changed as problems with this treatment emerged.

The Promise of Eternal Beauty and
Femininity: 1966–1975

Robert A. Wilson exemplifies physicians who made this promise when he wrote in *Feminine Forever*:

> I . . . believe that menopause prevention far transcends the purely clinical aspects of the subject. It even transcends any narrow view of sex as such. What is really at stake is a subtle and almost metaphysical factor—a woman's total femininity. (19)

Wilson, a Brooklyn gynecologist, was the most prolific and publicizing promoter of estrogen replacement therapy (ERT) in the 1960s. His research was well funded by the pharmaceutical industry since Ayerst Laboratories, Searle, and Upjohn supported the Wilson Research Foundation in New York City (Bruck; Johnson).

Feminine Forever, which sold 100,000 copies in the first seven months, was excerpted in *Vogue* and *Look* and discussed widely in the mass media. In the book, Wilson promised women that they could stay young and feminine forever and that menopause could be avoided completely. He labeled menopause a "hormone deficiency disease" and listed twenty-six symptoms—including absent-mindedness, irritability, depression, frigidity, alcoholism, and even suicide—that the "youth pill" could avert.

A number of prominent physicians, including William Masters (Johnson) and David Reuben, wrote popular articles claiming that ERT could stop aging, prevent cancer, and preserve sexuality. They frequently used Wilson as their primary or only source.

Addressing physicians, Robert Greenblatt, a former president of the American Geriatrics Society, supported Wilson by claiming that about seventy-five percent of menopausal women are estrogen deficient. He advocated ERT for these women even if they were without symptoms (Greenblatt). Some physicians, however, criticized Wilson's research methodology (Bruck), while others dismissed him as a quack, but rarely in public and always off the record (Seaman and Seaman).

Estrogen sales tripled from 1967 to 1975 (Seaman and Seaman). Women often asked their physicians to prescribe estrogen, since they were led to believe this "magic pill" could keep their skin smooth, their anger dampened, and their sex lives thriving. By 1975, Premarin, Ayerst's brand of estrogen, had become the fourth or fifth most popular drug in the United States—six million women were taking this medication (Seaman and Seaman). In the same year, a dramatic discovery led to the creation of a more modest promise.

The Promise of a Safe, Symptom-Free
Menopause: 1975–1981

Between 1975 and 1976, four papers published in the *New England Journal of Medicine* linked ERT to endometrial cancer (Smith et al.; Ziel and Finkle; Mack et al.; Weiss et al. 1976). After these reports, physicians thought twice before prescribing hormones for menopause. Prescriptions for ERT decreased by forty percent, with the greatest decline in high-dose products (Ernster et al.).

During this period, pharmaceutical companies selling estrogen emphasized, in their continuing marketing campaigns, the power of ERT to stop hot flashes, night sweating, and vaginal dryness. These physical changes were presented to women by physicians as symptoms requiring medical treatment (MacPherson 1981). The drug companies' claims were true, since ERT could eliminate these bodily changes. Then, as now, however, most women found simple ways—through self-help activities—to deal with these normal signs of menopause.

Misleading information circulated in the medical and lay literature that all women suffered at menopause, although earlier studies had clearly shown that this was not the case (McKinlay and McKinlay; McKinlay and Jefferys). Most women did not need ERT to stop hot flashes, night sweating, or vaginal dryness, since they were not particularly bothered by bodily changes that occurred at menopause. For these women, promises of being symptom free were not worth the risk of endometrial cancer. Thus, although certain claims for ERT were true, the promise that it was entirely safe was not.

The Promise of Escape from Chronic
Diseases: 1980–Present

The third promise given women was that hormones could prevent chronic diseases purportedly caused by menopause, such as osteoporosis and cardiovascular disease (CVD). Heretofore these conditions were related to aging. This new development coincided in 1981 with the birth of hormone replacement therapy (HRT).

The cancer scare of the mid-seventies was overcome by the addition of progestin, a synthetic progesterone, to the estrogen regimen. Usually a woman took estrogen twenty-five days and progestin five to fourteen days (Korenman 1982). Prescriptions for Provera, the most frequently prescribed progestin, grew steadily between 1980 and 1983.

Some physicians warned that caution was necessary, since the addition of progestin to estrogen could be tantamount to the use of oral contraceptives for the treatment of menopausal women (Wolff; Plunkett). Possible complications foreseen were gallbladder disease, thrombophlebitis, pulmonary embolus, stroke, myocardial infarction, or hypertension (Brenner). As the promises of preventing osteoporosis and cardiovascular disease have become more widely accepted, HRT prescriptions have continued to climb.

A current dominant medical trend is to link osteoporosis to menopause as a strongly contributing, if not the leading, causal factor (MacPherson 1987). Hormone replacement therapy is then presented as a logical and scientific choice to prevent or treat osteoporosis. Medical researchers point to the rapid loss of bone after bilateral oophorectomies if HRT is not given and compare this to the loss of bone after normal menopause (Aitken).

The promise of HRT for osteoporosis prevention needs careful scrutiny: Is it appropriate and ethical to give a potentially dangerous drug to healthy women as a preventive public health measure? Seventy-five percent of women will never have osteoporosis, yet many midlife women are routinely started on HRT by their physicians at menopause to prevent wrist, spinal, and hip fractures (National Institutes of Health). Once started on hormones, they must continue indefinitely or bone loss occurs at a rate similar to that seen immediately after menopause in women not given HRT (Lindsay et al.; Weiss et al.). Women taking HRT become dependent on expensive medical services—regular pelvic and breast exams, Pap smears, blood pressure monitoring, and endometrial biopsies.

Although HRT is widely prescribed for existing osteoporosis and has been approved by the Federal Drug Administration as a treatment, some bone experts believe that HRT does little for women who have low bone mass. These researchers report that HRT cannot restore bone mineral in elderly women with osteoporosis and therefore cannot reduce the fracture rate (Ettinger). It appears that when women already have osteoporosis, the most hormones can help to do is to keep bone mass at the level it was when HRT treatment was initiated.

Some studies have reported that estrogen replacement therapy also protects women against cardiovascular disease (CVD) (Adam et al.; Szklo et al.; Talbott et al.). Premature menopause has been identified as a serious risk for CVD. A large number of studies of disparate designs have been reasonably consistent in demonstrating that women with early bilateral oophorectomy are at risk and are helped by ERT (Stampfer et al.). Estrogen is, therefore, presumed to protect premenopausal women, and this protection is presumed to be lost after menopause when estrogen levels decline. Women who have experienced a natural menopause have not yet been subjects in substantive cardiovascular intervention research. Women were, however, included in the epidemiological research (known as the Framingham Study) that examined, over a twenty-four-year period, the factors that predispose people to develop CVD.

Cardiovascular disease has traditionally been viewed as primarily a male health problem, and most cardiovascular intervention studies have included only men as research subjects.

Yet CVD, including both heart disease and stroke, accounts for nearly fifty-three percent of all deaths in women over fifty years of age, compared to four percent of deaths due to breast cancer, eighteen percent caused by all other forms of cancer, and two percent resulting from accidents and suicides (National Center for Health Statistics). Heart disease and stroke are also a major cause of disability in older women. Even minor changes in risk for CVD could affect life expectancy in large numbers of women (Ernster et al.).

Traditional risk factors for CVD in women found in the biomedical literature include hypertension, cholesterol levels, smoking cigarettes, diabetes mellitus, excess weight, oral contraceptives, and genetics.

Hypertension

All types of CVD explored in the Framingham Study proved to be related to blood-pressure level. The strongest relationship was seen in atherothrombotic brain infarction and coronary heart disease (Dawber). In most published reports, an increase of 10 mm Hg in systolic blood pressure in women appears to be associated with a twenty to thirty percent risk of CVD death (Bush 1990). Hypertension is more prevalent in black compared to white women, and black women on antihypertensive medication seem to benefit more than white women in terms of fewer myocardial infarctions and strokes (Rosenthal).

Total Cholesterol, HDL Cholesterol, and
LDL Cholesterol

The Framingham Study provided convincing evidence that the overall level of cholesterol in the blood is a powerful factor in the development of CVD (Dawber). It was found that a low level of low-density lipoprotein fraction was positively related to CVD development, while high levels of high-density lipoproteins were negatively related.

An overview of research findings was presented at a recent National Conference on Cholesterol and High Blood Pressure Control by T. Bush, an epidemiologist. She reported that the level at which total cholesterol is a risk for women is not at 235 mg/dl, as for men, but at 265 mg/dl. In addition, there is some evidence that high total cholesterol is not as powerful a risk for women as for men. If HDL is high and total cholesterol is 264 mg/dl, a woman is not at high risk for CVD, but if HDL is low with total cholesterol of 264 mg/dl, a woman is at risk. She went on to say that safe LDL levels are not known, but that a combination of low HDL and high triglycerides are particularly lethal for women; women with a relatively low HDL and high triglycerides died 10 times the rate of women with relatively low triglycerides (Bush 1991). This report stressed that low HDL is a major predictor of CVD in women.

Smoking

Women who smoke one-half pack of cigarettes or one pack or more a day may have a fifty to one hundred percent increased risk of CVD death, respectively, compared to women who have never smoked (Bush and Comstock; Doll et al.). Smoking has also been implicated in women's experiencing an early menopause (Willet et al.).

Diabetes Mellitus

Diabetes Mellitus poses a serious threat for women developing CVD. In the Framingham Study, diabetes contributed substantially to the risk of all types of atherosclerotic disease: myocardial infarction, angina pectoris, peripheral arterial disease, and atherothrombotic stroke (Dawber).

Excess Weight

The Framingham Study also found that in all age categories, the evidence rate of CVD was fifty percent higher in people with greater relative weight. Body weight was firmly related to blood-pressure level; the magnitude of the weight–blood pressure relationship indicated that any attempt to lower blood pressure should involve weight reduction as a primary effort (Dawber). In contrast to women who smoke cigarettes and have an earlier than average menopause, heavier women tend to have menopause at a later age (Willett et al.).

Oral Contraceptives

Oral contraceptives contain synthetic estrogen and progesterone in doses high enough to prevent ovulation. Most studies have found that current use of oral contraceptives carries an increased risk of CVD in older premenopausal women who smoke cigarettes. Overall, it appears that there is not an increased risk of CVD among former oral contraceptive users (Barrett-Connor and Bush).

Genetics

It is reported to be a potent predictor of CVD in a woman if either of her parents have had a myocardial infarction prior to the age of sixty (Blackburn and Luepker).

Combination of Risk Factors

Each of the risk factors above has been found to increase the risk of CVD independently, and women with multiple risk factors have 10–12-fold increased risk of CVD (Gordon et al.).

Since 1952, nearly all studies confirm that oral estrogen causes lower low-density lipoprotein (LDL) and higher high-density lipoprotein (HDL) levels—a favorable ratio with regard to heart disease risk. LDL is often referred to as the "bad cholesterol," HDL as the "good cholesterol." On the one hand, estrogen suppresses formation of LDL, which carries cholesterol in the blood to the liver and to various other sites in the body. High levels of cholesterol-laden LDLs build up in the arterial walls, increasing risk of heart disease. On the other hand, estrogen enhances production of HDL, which scavenges cholesterol from the blood and the liver, then transports it to the intestines, where it is eliminated.

In a recent overview article, Barrett-Connor and Bush reviewed three studies that assessed the relationship between estrogen use and angiographically defined CVD in women. In all three reports women taking estrogen had significantly less artery stenosis than nonusers. There was a reported fifty-six to sixty-three percent reduction in risk of severe disease among users compared to nonusers.

The authors then summarized eighteen controlled observation studies assessing the effect of ERT on risk of CVD in women and stated that the majority of the reports found the reduction of risk ranged from forty-six to eighty-four percent and was independent of other known risk factors for CVD. Three studies found either no effect of noncontraceptive estrogen or a small reduction of risk for CVD. Four reports have found an increase in the risk of CVD among estrogen users.

A major new report (Stampfer et al.) on results of ERT use for both coronary disease and stroke is based on ten years of followup in the Nurses' Health Study. This was a large cohort research project that included 48,470 postmenopausal women. In those postmenopausal women who reported no previous CVD, the researchers documented 293 nonfatal myocardial infarctions and 112 deaths from coronary disease, as well as 172 nonfatal and 52 fatal strokes.

Overall, the age-adjusted risk of CVD morbidity or mortality among current ERT users was approximately half that of women who had never taken estrogen. The best supported finding in the study was the favorable effect of estrogen on cholesterol: estrogen raised the level of HDL and lowered the level of LDL.

Although the data appear persuasive for using ERT, the authors of the report gave several caveats. Estrogen users in the study were less likely to have diabetes, were lean, and were more likely to engage in regular, vigorous physical activity than nonusers. There was a nonsignificant trend in these data toward a decreasing benefit of estrogen with increasing age, which is consistent with the Framingham data. This merits close study in the future. If, in fact, this proves to be true, the argument for ERT could be weaker, since ERT would not have an impact on the prevention of CVD in older women, seventy and above, who clearly are at most risk. If there is a protective effect, it cannot protect women as they age, and the hypothesis is supported that CVD in women is primarily a disease of aging.

A serious problem with studies supporting the benefit of ERT is that all the major ones have involved estrogen regimens without progestin. *Right now the great unanswered question is whether a combination of estrogen and progestin is as protective against CVD as is estrogen alone.*

A large National Institutes of Health study called Postmenopausal Estrogen/Progestogen Intervention (PEPI), begun in the summer of 1989, is addressing the question of HRT and cardiovascular risk factors by including studies of blood clotting, blood pressure, and LDL and HDL levels. Bone loss and endometrial changes will also be monitored for the 840 women in the three-year study (National Women's Health Network; Barrett-Connor et al.). This is a limited intervention and the results will not be definitive. A long-term study of at least ten years' duration will be necessary to clearly determine whether estrogen combined with progestin can help to prevent CVD in postmenopausal women.

Although the false promises of HRT have been exposed, women will still face dilemmas in the 1990s as they hear conflicting reports about the potential benefits and potential risks of this "treatment" for menopause.

Current Dilemmas: Into the 1990s

Worries about endometrial cancer are still with us. The American Cancer Society has estimated that in 1987 there were 2,900 deaths and 35,000 new cases of endometrial cancer in the United States (Ernster et al.). There are no firm conclusions regarding the most effective progesterone and estrogen dosages. In addition, the breakthrough monthly bleeding for three to four days experienced by ninety-seven percent of women on HRT to help prevent endometrial cancer is objectionable to many women over sixty years of age. With ERT alone, however, bleeding is less predictable and potentially more problematic (Ernster et al.).

The relationship between HRT and breast cancer is still a vexing question today. Case studies conducted before 1980 were inconclusive. Since 1980 there have been ten case-controlled studies of ERT (Ernster et al.). Accumulated knowledge from these studies has been inconsistent and controversial. For example, a recent study in Uppsala, Sweden, involved 23,244 women who took hormones after menopause. The women were followed for an average of 5.7 years, and 253 of them developed breast cancer. One third of the women took progestin as well as estrogen. Among the women taking both drugs for four or more years, the rate of breast cancer was four times as high as the rate among women who took no hormones at all. Among women who took estrogen alone, the breast cancer rate was about double that of women who took no hormones (Bergkvist et al.). It is important to note that the Swedish women took a different form of estrogen than is used in the United States; this points to the need to replicate the study in this country with the commonly used form of estrogen.

American experts disagreed about whether the findings of this Swedish study, published in the *New England Journal of Medicine* (3 August, 1989), should cause women and their physicians to rethink their use of HRT (Kolata; Langone). Some gynecologists stated that the findings were inadequate to warrant a change in the current practice (Barrett-Connor). The possibility of increased risk of breast cancer has further muddled an already bewildering situation.

Using hormones to prevent or treat osteoporosis also poses dilemmas. HRT has to be continued indefinitely, some would argue from the start of menopause until death. As stated earlier, evidence suggests that much of the protective effect is lost within a few years of stopping HRT (Weiss et al. 1980). In addition, it is not clear if HRT is more or less effective than ERT for protection against bone loss. Studies done before 1986 looked at ERT for preventing osteoporosis. Whether HRT is more beneficial than ERT remains to be determined in long-term trials (Ernster et al.). Further, the optimal dose of estrogen for maximum benefit is uncertain; evidence is contradictory as to whether doses greater than 0.625 mg. per day offer more protection against fractures (Ernster et al.).

A final dilemma concerns hormonal treatment and heart disease. Unlike the positive effects of estrogen (ERT) when used alone, serum lipoproteins appear to be adversely affected by the addition of progestin. A variety of studies show HRT associated with an increase in LDL and a decrease in HDL (Barrett-Connor et al.). When progesterone is added to estrogen, its protective potential may disappear. Moreover, the addition of progesterone has been reported to increase total plasma cholesterol, and different dosages of progesterone produce different biological effects (Phillips).

Epidemiological studies need to be carried out to clarify the impact of progestins on estrogen's positive effect on cholesterol levels. To understand the CVD effects and the impact on breast cancer, these progestin studies should be carried on for at least ten years. A well-known researcher has stated: "If progestins must be given to prevent endometrial cancer, then the dose, duration, and frequency of therapy needs to be thoroughly assessed by a prospective controlled trial" (Korenman 1990, xv).

A major factor associated with prescribing progestins for post-menopausal women is that their natural progesterone levels are extremely low (Clark; Baird). Whereas lowered levels of estrogen continue to circulate in postmenopausal women until late in life, no research has been done that can explain what happens to older women's bodies over time when progestins are given. After menopause, they constitute an "untested hormonal experiment."

In 1988 an international consensus conference was organized to discuss the use of progestins following menopause (Whitehead and Lobo). There was consensus that because of lack of data, the use of progestins should be limited. It was also not recommended for hysterectomized women, as is sometimes advised, as a protection against breast cancer (Whitehead and Lobo).

A woman at risk for CVD with an intact uterus thus faces a painful dilemma—to choose a risk of endometrial cancer with estrogen alone to prevent CVD, or to take HRT without truly knowing what the long-term effect of progestin on CVD and on her body, in general, will be.

"Feminist distrust" is currently called for in analyzing the medical reductionist focus on cholesterol levels as the major risk factor for CVD in postmenopausal women and the "flaw in women's body" focus on postmenopausal estrogen "deficiency." Potent hormones given to healthy women, not to treat any disease, but to decrease potential of disease—specifically osteoporosis and CVD—from menopause until death seems like a reckless endeavor, since the risks of long-term use of HRT are not known at this time.

A major issue for feminists to study is the relationship between aging and CVD, which seems to be more supported by research data than the menopause–as–causation hypothesis. Unlike menopause, CVD occurs primarily in older women. This creates a serious time discordance between menopause and the disease, since ninety-five percent of women have undergone menopause by the age of fifty-five, and only less than one percent of women develop CVD by this age. Mortality rates for CVD do not approach one in one hundred until after age seventy. By this age the average woman has been postmenopausal for fifteen to twenty years (Perlman et al.). During this time, known risk factors combined with aging could play a large role in CVD morbidity or mortality.

Epidemiologists look upon menopause as a nondiscriminating variable in studies of women's health. This holds true with CVD, since currently there is no evidence from vital statistics data that natural menopause *per se* increases risk of CVD (Stampfer et al.; Bush 1990).

Known risk factors, such as family history, smoking, hypertension, diabetes, high cholesterol, and oral contraceptives, are reported to be so predictive that they overwhelm the hypothesis of causation related to menopause alone (Dawber). The highest single predictor of future CVD has been identified as hypertension (Blackburn and Luepker).

Health care providers can be helpful by reviewing each risk factor or multiple risk factors with a woman on an individual basis and constructing with her a plan for any beneficial changes that is realistic, acceptable, and economically viable. Women who experience an early natural or surgical menopause need special, highly individual attention regarding the issues

156   The Hormone Replacement Therapy Debate

surrounding ERT and HRT in order to make informed choices that they
feel good about.

Women themselves can turn to self-help literature for steps they can
take to reduce their risks for CVD, such as regular exercise and a low-fat
diet, as well as for balanced information about the HRT dilemma (Doress
and Siegal; Cobb). Two research-based books by a physician give clear
guidance on how to prevent CVD and how it can be reversed (Ornish
1982, 1990).

The three false promises given to women over the years about the safe
and positive effects of ERT and HRT were built upon the medical ideology of menopause as a disease requiring hormonal intervention. As we
move into the 1990s, the raging debate over the potential benefits and
risks of HRT (which is rooted in conflicting research findings) do little to
solve the dilemmas women face. One thing is certain—women should inform themselves as thoroughly as possible before accepting HRT.

REFERENCES

Adam, S.; Williams, V.; and Vessey, M. P. (1981). Cardiovascular disease and hor-
    mone replacement treatment: A pilot case-control study. *British Medical
    Journal* 282, 1277–78.
Aitken, J. M. (1973). Oestrogen replacement therapy for prevention of osteoporo-
    sis after oophorectomy. *British Medical Journal* 3, 515ff.
Baird, B. (1978). Patterns of sex hormone production in women. In Oliver, M.
    (ed.). *Coronary Heart Disease in Young Women*. New York: Longman.
Barrett-Connor, E. (1989). Postmenopausal estrogen replacement and breast can-
    cer. *New England Journal of Medicine* 321, 319.
Barrett-Connor, E., and Bush, T. (1991). Estrogen and coronary heart disease in
    women. *Journal American Medical Association* 265 (14), 1861–66.
Barrett-Connor, E.; Wingard, D,; and Criqui, M. (1989). Postmenopausal estrogen
    use and heart disease risk factors in the 1980s. *Journal American Medical
    Association* 261 (14), 2095–99.
Bell, S. E. (1980). The synthetic compound diethylstilbestrol (DES) 1938–1941:
    The social construction of a medical treatment. Doctoral thesis. Brandeis
    University, Waltham, Mass.
Bergkvist, L.; Hans-Olov, A.; Persson, I.; Hoover, R.; and Schairer, C. (1989). The
    risk of breast cancer after estrogen and estrogen-progestin replacement.
    New England Journal of Medicine 321, 293–97.
Blackburn, H., and Luepker, R. (1987). Heart disease. In Last, J. (ed.). *Preventive
    Medicine and Public Health*. New York: Medical Publishers. Chap. 3.
Brenner, P. (1982). The menopause (Medical Progress). *Western Journal of Medi-
    cine* 136, 211–19.
Bruck, C. (1979). Menopause. *Human Behavior* 8 (4), 38–46.

Bush, T. (1990). Epidemiology of cardiovascular disease. *Annals of the New York Academy of Sciences* 592, 263–71.

———. (1991). Women and cardiovascular disease. Paper presented at the National Conference on Cholesterol and High Blood Pressure Control. Washington, D.C. 8–10 April.

Bush, T., and Comstock, G. (1983). Smoking and cardiovascular mortality in women. *American Journal of Epidemiology* 118, 480–88.

Clark, J. (1990). Actions of estrogen: Molecule, biological and evolutionary considerations. In Korenman, S. (ed.). *The Menopause.* Norwell, Mass.: Serono Symposia.

Cobb, J. L. (1991). Estrogen, breast cancer, heart disease. *A Friend Indeed* viii (8), 1–4.

Dawber, T. (1980). *The Framingham Study.* Cambridge: Harvard University Press.

Doll, R.; Gray, R.; Hafner, G.; et al. (1980). Mortality in relation to smoking: 22 years' observation on female British doctors. *British Medical Journal* 1, 967–71.

Doress, P., and Siegal, D. (1987). *Ourselves, Growing Older: Women Aging with Knowledge and Power.* New York: Simon and Schuster.

Ernster, V.; Bush, T.; Huggins, G.; Hulka, B.; Kelsey, J.; and Schottenfeld, D. (1988). Clinical perspectives: Benefits and risks of menopausal estrogen and/or progestin hormone use. *Preventive Medicine* 17, 201–23.

Ettinger, B. (1987). Postmenopausal bone loss is prevented by treatment with low-dosage estrogen with calcium. *Annals of Internal Medicine* 106, 40–45.

Gordon, T.; Kannel, W.; and Hjortland, M. (1978). Menopause and coronary heart disease: The Framingham Study. *Annals of Internal Medicine* 89, 157–61.

Greenblatt, R. (1974). *The Menopausal Syndrome.* New York: Medcom.

Hubbard, R., and Lowe, M. (1983). *Women's Nature: Rationalizations of Inequality.* New York: Pergamon.

Johnson, A. (1977). The risk of sex hormones as drugs. *Women and Health* 2 (1), 8–11.

Kolata, G. (1989). Menopause hormone linked to breast cancer. *New York Times,* 3 Aug. 1, B6.

Korenman, S. (1982). Menopausal endocrinology and management. *Archives of Internal Medicine* 142, 1131–36.

———. (1990) (ed). *The Menopause.* Norwell, Mass.: Serono Symposia.

Langone, J. (1989). Hard look at hormones: Drugs to ease the toll of menopause are linked to breast cancer. *TIME,* 14 Aug. 56.

Lindsay, R.; Hart, D.; McLean, A.; Clark, A.; Kraszewski, A.; and Garwood, J. (1978). Bone response to termination of estrogen treatment. *Lancet* 1, 1325–27.

Mack, T.; Pike, M.; Henderson, B.; Pfeffer, R.; Gerkins, V.; Arthur, M.; and Brown, S. (1976). Estrogens and endometrial cancer in a retirement community. *New England Journal of Medicine* 294, 1262–67.

MacPherson, K. I. (1981). Menopause as disease: The social construction of a metaphor. *Advances in Nursing Science* 3 (2), 95–113.

———. (1987). Osteoporosis: The new flaw in woman or in science? *Health Values* 11 (4), 57–62.

McKinlay, S., and Jefferys, M. (1974). The Menopausal Syndrome. *British Journal of Preventive Social Medicine* 28 (2), 108–15.

McKinlay, S. M., and McKinlay, J. B. (1973). Selected studies of the menopause. *Journal Biosocial Science* 5, 533–55.

National Center for Health Statistics (1986). *Vital Statistics of the United States.* Vol II. Mortality, Parts A and B. Pub. No. (DHHS) 88–1122 and 88–1114. Washington, D.C.: Public Health Service.

National Institutes of Health (1984). Osteoporosis: Consensus Development Conference Statement. Bethesda, Md.: NIH.

National Women's Health Network (1989). Taking hormones and health: Choices, risks, benefits. Washington, D.C.: National Women's Health Network.

Ornish, D. (1982). *Stress, diet and your heart.* New York: Holt, Rinehart and Winston.

———. (1990). *Dr. Dean Ornish's program for reversing heart disease.* New York: Random House.

Perlman, J.; Wolf, P.; Finucane, F.; and Madans, J. (1989). Menopause and the epidemiology of cardiovascular disease in women. *Progress in Clinical and Biological Research* 320, 283–312.

Phillips, P. (1988). Progestogen sets lipid profiles. *Medical World News* 25 April. 80.

Plunkett, E. R. (1982). Contraceptive steroids, age and the cardiovascular system. *American Journal of Obstetrics and Gynecology* 142 (6), 747–51.

Reinharz, S. (1985). Feminist distrust: Problems of context and content in sociological work. In Berg D. N. and Smith K. D. (eds.). *Exploring Clinical Methods for Social Research.* Beverly Hills, Calif.: Sage. 153–72.

Reuben, D. (1969). *Everything you always wanted to know about sex.* New York: Bantam.

Rosenthal, E. (1989). Different but deadly. *New York Times Magazine* 17 September. 120–21.

Schiff, T. (1979). Risks and benefits of estrogen use. Presented at the NIH Consensus Development Conference on Estrogen Use. Washington, D.C. September.

Seaman, B., and Seaman, G. (1977). *Women and the crisis in sex hormones.* New York: Bantam.

Smith, D.; Pentice, A.; Donovan, J.; and Herrmann, W. (1975). Association of exogenous estrogen and endometrial carcinoma. *New England Journal of Medicine* 293, 1164–67.

Stampfer, M.; Colditz, G.; Willett, W.; Manson, J.; Rosner, B.; Speizer, F.; et al. (1991). Postmenopausal estrogen therapy and cardiovascular disease. *New England Journal of Medicine* 325, 756–62.

Szklo, M.; Tonascia, J.; Gordis, L.; and Bloom, I. (1984). Estrogen use and myocardial infarction risk: A case-control study. *Preventive Medicine* 13, 510–16.

Talbot, E.; Kuller, L. II.; and Detre, K. (1977). Biologic and psychosocial risk factors of sudden death from coronary disease in white women. *American Journal of Cardiology* 39, 858–64.

Weiss, N.; Szekely, D.; and Austin, F. (1976). Increasing incidence of endometrial cancer in the U.S. *New England Journal of Medicine* 294, 1259–62.

Weiss, N.; Ure, C.; Ballard, J.; Williams A.; and Daling, J. (1980). Decreased risk of fractures of the hip and lower forearm with postmenopausal use of estrogen. *New England Journal of Medicine* 303, 1195–98.

Whitehead, M., and Lobo, R. (1988). Progestin use in postmenopausal women. *Lancet* i, 1243–44.

Willett, W.; Stampfer, M.; Bain, C.; et al. (1983). Cigarette smoking, relative weight, and menopause. *American Journal of Epidemiology* 117, 651–58.

Wilson, R. A. (1966). *Feminine forever.* New York: M. Evans.

Wolff, S. (1984). Statement of public citizens group. Read before the National

Institutes of Health Consensus Development Conference on Osteoporosis. Bethesda, Md. 14 April.

Ziel, H., and Finkle, W. (1975). Increased risk of endometrial carcinoma among users of conjugated estrogens. *New England Journal of Medicine* 293, 1167–70.

Zola, I. K. (1972). Medicine as an institution of social control. *Sociology Review* 20, 487–504.

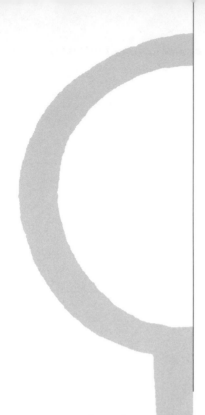

A Journey to the Center of the Cell: Understanding the Physiology and Endocrinology of Menopause

Ann M. Voda

Introduction: Another Fine Myth You've Gotten Us Into

Menstruating women cause dryness in milk cows and can kill a young fruit tree. When such events occur the offending woman is to be tortured, put to flame, and burned at the stake (Delaney et al.). Women are to be drugged and sometimes institutionalized because of affective or somatic changes at menopause (MacPherson 1981). Only a few years ago these were prevalent American beliefs. Ridiculous, now. Horrifying, even then. Never again, we are certain.

Today such notions seem merely folk tales of a bygone era. We are modern, thinking beings and have been saved from folly and fallacy by modern medicine. We have replaced the imaginings of myth-makers with the objectivity of scientists. Think again. That equally absurd and culpable mythologies persist is well documented. They are the new myths for the 1990s. They are more dangerous and pervasive than any that have come before, threatening the well-being of millions of women in the United States and millions more throughout the world (Golub; Asso; Delaney et al.; Fausto-Sterling; Taylor; Lander; Dan et al.; Komnenich et al; Cutler; Voda 1980, 1981a; Voda et al. 1982).

What are these new myths? The prescription of steroid sex hormones

for healthy women to prevent pregnancy, heart attacks, spine and hip fractures, and breast cancer, bolstered by claims that the beneficial effects of
these substances outweigh their risks, tops the list.

Hormone Myth One: From Crocodile Dung to Steroid Hormones

In our lifetime, scientific discoveries have vastly improved the conditions and quality of life. Certain advances in contraceptive technology
now permit women to be as sexually free as men without fear of pregnancy and to control family planning in ways only dreamed of several
decades ago. Oral contraceptives, combinations of estrogen and progester-
one-like sex steroids, represent modern-day scientific contributions to the
unending search for the ideal contraceptive. This particular method of
contraception represents a dramatic breakaway from older, culturally specific methods of birth control ranging from pessaries made of crocodile
dung to diaphragms and spermicidal jellies, and from potions of quick-
silver and oil to eating the uterus of a female mule (Kistner).

These methods seem crude, and we expect folk trial and error and
untested potions, medicines, and devices to be eliminated from an advanced society. Dangerous substances would be recognized, and no
healthy individual would be expected to take a drug or use a device once
its potential to harm was known (Voda 1981a). Yet, women remain in
harm's way.

Currently 13.8 million women in the United States and 60 million
worldwide use steroidal oral contraceptives for birth control (Hatcher et
al.). The first concerns over the safety and health risks to women using
these drugs were raised in the mid-1970s. Widespread use of oral contraceptives prompted Hellman, then newly elected president of the American
Gynecological Society, in his 1975 keynote address to suggest that a therapeutic dilemma has reared its head in medicine: For the first time in re-
corded history, healthy people are taking potent drugs voluntarily over a
long period for an objective other than controlling disease (Hellman). The
"well" people Hellman referred to were young women of reproductive
age. Since then hormone usage has doubled (Hatcher et al.).

The first warnings emerged from the United Kingdom, where an increased risk of heart attack and circulatory problems was reported as occurring in 46,000 women using oral contraceptives (Beral 1977). This
study, which reported on 200,000 women-years of "pill" use, suggested

that the difference in death rate from diseases of the circulatory system between those who have at any time used oral contraceptives and those who have never done so was 20 per 100,000 women per year, an increase of one death per 5,000 oral contraceptive users per year (Beral 1976, 1977). Advocates of the hormone method of contraception maintained that risks connected with its use were small and insignificant compared with the risks associated with pregnancy. Based upon this risk/benefit analysis, oral contraceptives were and are declared extremely safe for young women, even though a variety of disadvantages are associated with their use (Hatcher et al.). For example, after more than two decades of oral contraceptive use, circulatory disorders, identified in the 1970s as serious complications, are just as risky for women in the 1990s, with the risk increasing in women users older than thirty-five who smoke (Beral 1976, 1977; Hatcher et al.).

Whether or not the hormone-like drugs contained in oral contraceptives cause cancer has been a source of continuing debate, particularly because of the long latency period that is possible between exposure to a carcinogen and clinical manifestations of cancer. An example of the temporal aspects of cancer latency tragically surfaced years after some women in the 1940s and 1950s took the drug diethylstilbestrol (DES), a nonsteroidal synthetic estrogen-like compound, to prevent miscarriages. Women exposed to the drug while in their mothers' wombs have ten to twenty years later developed cancer of the vagina, miscarried when pregnant, experienced ectopic (out of womb) pregnancies, and/or birthed premature babies (Hatcher et al.). Another example of latency between carcinogen and clinical appearance of cancer is an increased rate of breast cancer in the women who took DES to prevent miscarrying. Twenty years had to elapse before the rate of breast cancer was observed to increase in these women (Greenberg et al.).

As the twenty-first century rushes toward us, proponents of steroidal methods of contraception are very excited about six new progestin-only approaches to birth control. These methods offer protection from pregnancy from three months, via injection of Depo-Provera, to up to five years with the new implant, Norplant. Norplant involves a minor surgical implantation of small silicone tubes beneath the surface of the skin. These tubes contain the progestin Levonorgestrel, which is periodically diffused into the body (Hatcher et al.).

It is unknown whether breast cancer will be latently expressed in any specific group of women using steroidal contraceptives, such as the progestin-only users, users prior to first-term pregnancy, users with fibrocystic breast disease, steroidal contraceptive users whose breast cancer is diagnosed at a young age or premenopausally, and long-term steroidal contraceptive users (Hatcher et al.). It is known that during the almost three decades of oral contraceptive use, the incidence of breast cancer in general has increased steadily, with the most dramatic increase occurring over the last three years, from one in fourteen to one in nine women (American Cancer Society).

Hormone Myth Two: From Menopausal Estrogen Deficiency to Climacteric Endocrinopathy

In 1963 Robert Wilson, a New York gynecologist, gave birth to the myth of menopause as an estrogen deficiency disease. Despite scientific advancements and sophistication in research methods, Wilson's negative view of menopause established an ideology and a medical following that has gained momentum over the past thirty years. Wilson believed that without estrogen replacement a woman's postmenopausal destiny was to spend the rest of her life in living decay (Wilson and Wilson). So powerful and convincing were his arguments in favor of estrogen replacement that in the 1970s estrogen hormone in the form of estrone (F_1) was one of the top five prescriptions sold in the United States (National Women's Health Network). Estimations of hormone use at this time suggested that one-third of women over age fifty were using it regularly (Stadel and Weiss).

Estrogen was promoted as a wonder drug. The benefits promised for menopausal women who used it would be to age more slowly, be sexually attractive, and avoid the psychological problems associated with menopause (National Women's Health Network). Wilson also proclaimed that the hormone would protect against osteoporosis, heart disease, and cancers of the breast and uterus. Risks to health were minimized. In his book *Feminine Forever*, which sold over 100,000 copies in seven months (Seaman and Seaman), Wilson painted a compelling word picture of the horrors of a woman's living her postmenopausal years in a body without estrogen—a body that would ultimately betray her through crushing fractures, a dried, cracked, and bleeding vagina, clogged arteries, and unbearable hot flashes (MacPherson 1981).

In the mid-1970s, the myth of estrogen forever/ feminine forever/ healthy forever was exposed when several epidemiological studies linked postmenopausal estrogen use to endometrial hyperplasia (buildup of uterine endometrium) and adenocarcinoma (cancer) (Smith et al.; Ziel and Finkle; Mack et al.).

In 1984 an estimated 39,000 cases of endometrial carcinoma were reported and 2,900 deaths from the disease were reported (Silverberg). Following the publicity about the estrogen/cancer connection, widespread treatment of menopausal women diminished, and estrogen prescriptions decreased by forty percent (MacPherson 1991). From 1975 to 1980, a concerted effort to rehabilitate estrogen therapy was undertaken. A major step toward rehabilitation resulted when a progestin (a steroid compound related to progesterone) was added to the estrogen that women were taking in pill form (National Women's Health Network).

Progesterone is a female sex hormone synthesized normally during the postovulatory phase of the menstrual cycle. A major metabolic function of progesterone during the menstrual cycle is to transform the uterine endometrium, which proliferates rapidly under the influence of estrogens, into a secretory organ. If conception occurs, this transformation is necessary for implantation of the developing ball of cells, the blastocyst. In technical terms, progesterone antagonizes estrogen's powerful proliferative (mitotic) cell division effect on the uterine endometrium (Schenken and Pauerstein).

In the 1980s estrogen replacement therapy for a pre- or postmenopausal woman with a uterus became hormone replacement therapy, the combination of estrogen and a progestin. This change in hormone therapy was quickly accepted by physicians and recommended by the American College of Obstetrics and Gynecology (Barrett-Connor 1987). Seaman's concern in 1975 over the experimental nature of oral contraceptives remained unheard in the 1980s as another drug regimen for use in healthy women became widely accepted with little critical study (Barrett-Connor 1987). The establishment of menopause as disease was completed when the link between osteoporosis (demineralization of bone) and estrogen deficiency was made explicit and when the beneficial effects of estrogens in reducing heart disease in women received medical endorsement (MacPherson 1985; Barrett-Connor 1987). So eager was the crowd to join the parade that few bothered to consider that these links and endorsements were used to form erroneous conclusions.

Thirty years later, Wilson's estrogen forever/feminine forever myth has been partly dismantled insofar as estrogen has been identified as being very risky for a woman with a uterus. Nevertheless, replacement therapy in the 1990s is grounded in Wilson's basic premise that menopause is a disease. Fifteen years beyond the establishment of the causal link between uterine cancer and estrogen, the debate no longer is whether menopausal women should take estrogen; rather, the questions have become: For what disease prevention should estrogen be prescribed? and What is the safest way to administer the hormone? A major difference between Wilson and modern-day clinicians is that menopause per se is not taken as the disease to be treated; instead, treatment is thought to be necessary to prevent the debilitating effects of certain diseases, most notably osteoporosis and coronary artery disease, which are postulated to occur as a result of a climacteric-related endocrinopathy (Utian 1990).

Evidence to support the climacteric as an endocrinopathy is based upon the demonstration of four classical sequential steps: (1) a morphological change in the ovary, which is an endocrine gland, (2) an alteration in the endocrine milieu, that is, changes in sex-hormone concentrations, (3) changes in receptor target tissue, such as urogenital tissue, in response to changes in hormone levels, and, (4) the presentation to clinicians of women with complaints as a result of changes in endocrine glands, target tissues, and hormone levels (Utian 1990).

Utian (1987) argued that the nature of these changes justified some form of hormone replacement in appropriately selected women. What makes Utian's view of menopause important for women is that it comes from a source we want to trust. Wulf Utian is the president of the North American Menopause Society as well as the president-elect of the International Menopause Society. His definition of the climacteric as endocrinopathy was constructed to represent a subset of women in whom certain changes were viewed as outside of the context of normality. Whether or not this definition will be appropriately applied or taken out of context remains to be seen. Most clinicians, despite Utian's attempts to bring about more precision in medical diagnosis, will associate menopause and midlife in women with estrogen deficiency.

The definition of menopause as disease or as endocrinopathy has its origins in patriarchal views and beliefs about women as defective, imperfect, or as machines that need to be fixed (Martin). This damning perspective on menopause permeates society, science, and medical practice and has eclipsed the view of menopause as a normal biological event (MacPherson 1981, 1985; Voda and Eliasson; Voda and George).

Biology Is Destiny: Hormones and Change

For almost one-half of her life a woman experiences constant changes resulting from cyclic fluctuations in a variety of peptide and steroid sex hormones. Estrogen and progesterone are the primary sex steroid hormones synthesized by the ovaries. During reproductive years, menarche through menopause, the concentration of these hormones in the blood rises and falls with the phases of the menstrual cycle.

During prime reproductive years, the dominant estrogen in a woman's body is 17 Beta estradiol (E_2), which initiates the process of building up the uterine lining during the follicular phase of her cycle. Under the influence of E_2, uterine cells line up and divide, and the uterine endometrium becomes hyperplastic. On or around day thirteen, there is an estradiol surge, a precipitous increase in and peak of E_2, which is followed immediately by a peak (surge) of luteotrophic hormone (LH) from the brain. The occurrence of these two events within precise temporal parameters is followed by ovulation, that is, the extrusion of an ovum from an ovarian follicle.

Following ovulation, the concentration of LH decreases and E_2 begins to rise. The postovulatory phase of the cycle is referred to as the luteal phase and is characterized by progesterone synthesis. Luteal-phase estrogen regulates the synthesis of receptors for progesterone. During this phase of the cycle, progesterone stops the uterine cells from dividing and, via a process called differentiation, transforms the uterine cells into cells which perform specialized functions necessary to sustain pregnancy. In other words, cell differentiation transforms the uterus into a very hospitable environment for the blastocyst to implant and continue growth to embryo and fetus. If no sperm is available to fuse with an egg, there is no pregnancy, and on about day twenty-three or twenty-four, estrogen and progesterone levels fall. Menstruation, the process of shedding the uterine endometrium, begins around day twenty-six to twenty-eight of the menstrual cycle. As menstruation occurs, the concentration of estradiol increases and the entire process begins again (Voda 1981a).

As the concentration of estradiol and progesterone fluctuates during menstrual-cycle phases, women experience somatic changes such as water retention, bloating, breast tenderness, appetite and energy changes, and affective changes, such as irritability and mood changes (Voda 1980). These changes are hormonally mediated and are signs that the necessary physiological and biochemical adjustments have been made to ensure a successful blastocyst implantation into the uterus (Voda and Randall). Rather than viewing these menstrual-cycle changes as normal in preparation for pregnancy, they have been conceptualized within a pathophysiological paradigm, namely, premenstrual syndrome (PMS).

It is now an understatement to say that considerable attention has been given to the study of psychophysiological aspects of the menstrual cycle.

Clinical or medical interest in menstrual-cycle physiology was at first generated by the varied complaints women presented to their physicians during the premenstruum. These complaints, initially referred to as premenstrual distress (Frank), are now referred to as PMS (Keye). Fluctuating gonadal hormones, estrogen and progesterone, are thought to cause the physical and psychological distress experienced by women. The exact mechanism by which they cause PMS remains unclear and, unfortunately, a demand for care and treatment has come before a thorough understanding of PMS has been reached (Keye).

The biomedical model of PMS has its origin deeply rooted in Frank's model of premenstrual tension. What contemporary physicians overlooked in Frank's model was the reference to normal women. According to Frank, it was known that many women experienced varying degrees of discomfort preceding the onset of menstruation. However, these discomforts were viewed as normal. Like Utian's definition of climacteric endocrinopathy, it was outside of the context of normalcy in which Frank identified a class of patients in whom grave systemic disorders were manifest during the premenstrual period. These women, according to Frank, were experiencing severe premenstrual tension. Since the resurrection of Frank's model of premenstrual tension in 1982, the legacy from more than a decade of publicity and media hype on PMS has revived old stereotypes about women as sick, hysterical, victims of their hormones, and that biology is destiny for illness or disease. In short, the PMS woman has emerged as the prototype for all menstruating women in the 1990s.

Sex Hormones as Metabolic Regulators

Too few women understand what they need to know about how sex hormones function; nor do they understand basic biological processes well enough to appreciate that on the one hand the changes that occur in their bodies are, on average, normal, whether during the menstrual cycle, pregnancy, or menopause, and, on the other hand, are a result of fluctuating levels of steroid sex hormones.

Hormones. Hormones, in general, are part of the body's regulatory system. They are the wireless counterpart of the nervous system. Hormones function according to a basic physiological law of supply and demand. Very simply, when the stimulus to conserve, pump, or utilize water, sodium, calcium, phosphorous, or glucose is received, the demand is met partially by feedback relationships between these substances and the gland that secretes a specific regulatory hormone. In other situations (such as thyroid secretion, cortisol secretion, and in the regulation of reproductive physiology) there is a dynamic state of hormone balance based on the principle of negative feedback.

A few concepts are important to the understanding of how hormones work in the body and how they regulate metabolism.

First, hormones are metabolic regulators. They do not initiate action; rather, they increase or decrease basal metabolic processes. The ability to just maintain or, more specifically, to function at a basal level is present in all cells. When a demand is placed upon an individual and there is a need to increase metabolism, hormones are secreted into the circulation, where they bind with cellular receptors in target tissue.

Second, the concentration of free hormone in the blood is very low. In the case of the sex steroids, estrogen and progesterone, circulating blood concentrations are extremely low, for example, in picogram (10 to the minus 12th gram) amounts for estrogen and nanogram (10 to the minus 9th gram) concentrations for progesterone. Hormones are degraded continuously; synthesis is a complex relationship of free hormone, degradative capacity, and feedback demand for its regulatory function.

Third, hormones are classified mainly as peptides, proteins, amines, prostaglandins, or steroids. At the cellular level they differ in mechanism of action depending on their classification and chemical makeup.

Fourth, hormones regulate metabolism indirectly via a process called "receptor mediated signal transduction." Protein, peptide, and amine hormones regulate cell metabolism by interacting with receptors on target cell membranes. However, steroid hormones, because they are lipid in nature, diffuse freely through membranes of all cells. In target cells, particularly genitourinary cells, steroids bind with receptors inside the cell.

Steroid Hormones. The most important steroid hormones are the sex steroid hormones, progesterone and estradiol, the adrenal steroids, cortisol and aldosterone, the androgenic hormone testosterone, and vitamin D$_3$. All steroids perform different functions in the body. To understand the many side effects associated with taking steroids, several concepts specific to steroid hormones need to be understood.

First, all steroids are structurally similar. All have the basic four-ring structure of cholesterol as common building material. The different functions of steroids are attributable to the way in which side groups are attached to the four-ring molecule.

Second, steroids bind first with intracellular (cytosolic) receptors in target tissue. In uterine and breast cells, for example, the process of binding creates a new compound, a hormone-receptor-complex. This complex translocates, moving into the nucleus where it attaches to certain proteins on deoxyribonucleic acid (DNA), namely, the chromatin material or the genome (O'Malley and Schrader; Voda 1981a).

Third, after nuclear binding, steroids stimulate the synthesis of proteins that increase or decrease metabolism, enzymes, receptors for hormones, growth factors, and so on.

During the follicular phase of the menstrual cycle, the genetic message transcribed via estrogen hormone-receptor binding onto DNA is to promote uterine cell proliferation. Following ovulation during the luteal phase of the cycle, the progesterone-hormone-complex binding with DNA initiates protein synthesis, which stops cell division. This process is enhanced by enzymes that change the structure and function of the endometrial cells.

Fourth, and as already mentioned, steroids are present in the blood in very low concentrations. The unbound or free concentration of estradiol during menstrual years is in picogram amounts. Progesterone concentrations during the luteal phase of the cycle can reach 10 nanograms or more. Substances found in oral contraceptives are prescribed in micrograms. (A microgram is 10^{-6} gram.) For example, thirty-five micrograms of ethinyl estradiol found in the birth control pill is greater than the naturally synthesized concentration of picogram quantities of estradiol found in the blood. The daily dose of estrogen (Estrone) prescribed for postmenopausal women is in milligram quantities, which is, theoretically, *more than a million times the concentration of natural estrogens*. Progesterone replacement at menopause in the form of medroxyprogesterone acetate (MPA) is prescribed in ten-milligram quantities. *This dose is one million times greater than the concentration of progesterone measured in the blood.*

The side effects associated with sex steroid use (whether for contraception or menopausal replacement) are a result of two factors. One, the dosages of hormones prescribed are not physiological. They are pharmacological. Two, even though the affinity for estrogen to bind with receptors for other steroids (such as the receptors for cortisol and/or aldosterone) is low, because the estrogens are administered in pharmacological concentrations greater than those normally found in the body and because all steroids are structurally similar, they are able to bind with receptors for other steroids and turn them on. That is, they activate the DNA in cells other than those in reproductive target tissue.

The compounds found in oral contraceptives provide an example. The estrogen-like substances commonly used in the pill are ethinyl estradiol

and mestranol. Unlike the natural hormone, estradiol, these two substances, while resembling estrogen, are not the same as the substances
synthesized in the body. They are drugs. Both ethinyl estradiol and mestranol have an ethinyl side group attached to the carbon 17 position on the
four-membered cholesterol skeleton. In addition, mestranol has a methyl
ether at the third carbon position. These modifications of the natural hormone are necessary in order to prevent metabolic inactivation in the gas-
trointestinal tract. As the drugs in oral contraceptives are absorbed, the
liver is the first organ to be presented with a bolus, a large volume, of
steroid-like drug. Here the probability for the compounds to bind with
cortisol receptors is high. Binding results in the synthesis of proteins that
promote gluconeogenesis (synthesis of glucose from protein), which is
manifested clinically as a prediabetic condition. Binding may also result in
an increase in the synthesis of live enzymes that promote clotting and
increases cardiovascular risks associated with sex steroid use, such as
stroke. Most of the side effects listed in patient package inserts are related
to the ability of sex steroids to bind with receptors, mimicking the action
of other steroids. At times, however, binding may produce an antagonistic
effect, for example, blocking the hormone's action. This creates the possibility for increased risk of heart disease for menopausal women with a
uterus when progesterone is added to estrogen.

Closure of Menstrual Life

After thirty-five to thirty-seven years of menstrual life, which has been
dominated by fluctuating levels of sex steroid hormones, turning on and
turning off metabolic processes in reproductive tissue, a woman's capacity
to reproduce diminishes and menstruation ceases. The genetic message to
terminate reproductive capacity around age fifty was preprogrammed
while the woman was a fetus developing in her mother's womb. For unknown reasons, at menopause ovarian tissue becomes less and less respon-
sive to brain hormones. Subsequently, steroid hormone synthesis
decreases, menstrual cycles become anovulatory, and after a period of irregular menstruations, which may be characterized by either or both long
and short intervals between bleeds (Treloar et al.) and/or heavy bleeding
and passing of clots (Voda and Mansfield in progress), menstruation stops.
Menopause has arrived.

As transition to menopause begins, certain changes occur. Some or all
may occur well in advance of any change in bleeding pattern and may

persist for years after the last bleed. There begins an almost imperceptible estrogen and progesterone decline. There may be an increase in the variability of bleeds and intermenstrual intervals. There may be no indicators other than the perception that subtle changes have begun.

Sporadic ovarian synthesis of estradiol results in a continuous decline of the hormone, and as estrogen levels decline, so does progesterone. Menopause may be due to irregular maturation of residual follicles and/or diminished responsiveness to gonadotrophin or brain stimulation (Korenman et al.). The number of follicles in an ovary begins to decline around the twentieth week of gestation (Bloch). This decrease steadily continues until menopause, when the ovary has been described as depleted of follicles (Utian 1987).

Women and their care providers frequently have no overt indication or index to use to monitor for subtle changes. Neither vaginal smears nor endometrial biopsies give any indication of the dynamics of entry into the transition. However, the closure of reproductive years is a dynamic process, a period of hormone fluctuations and change. As such, the static understanding of menopause as the last menstrual bleed needs to be differentiated from several other concepts:

Menopausal Transition. A period of time marked by progressive change in the pattern of menstrual bleeding, terminating at menopause. The pattern may be one of unusually long or short intervals between bleeds, accompanied by bleeding which is heavy and gushing and/or with clots (Treloar et al.; Voda and Mansfield in progress).

Perimenopausal Transition. By definition, this is the onset of a somatic change, such as hot flash, which may precede the change in menstrual bleeding pattern but which persists throughout the climacteric into the postmenopausal years (Voda and George).

Menopause. The clinical definition of menopause is the cessation of menstruation at the last menstrual bleed. It is affirmed after one year has elapsed from the last menstrual bleed. Should a woman experience another bleed at any time, her menopause would then be considered to be at what subsequently becomes her last menstrual bleed. However, the widespread use of steroid sex hormones, either for contraception or to "treat" menopause, and the implementation of aggressive treatment modalities—surgery, radiation and chemotherapy—for some diseases, such as cancer, has necessitated expanding the definition of menopause to differentiate between menopause as a natural occurrence from menopause that has been induced or effected by either surgery, hormone usage, or radiation and chemotherapy.

Natural menopause is the final spontaneous menstrual bleed. It most commonly occurs around age fifty. It occurs only in women who have retained their ovaries and who have not taken estrogen, either in birth control pills or through estrogen replacement.

Hormonal menopause occurs in any woman who has ever been a sex hormone user. Hormone use includes use of the estrogens (e.g., estrone, estradiol), progestins (e.g., MPA, Norgesterol, Norethindrone), and the estrogen- and progestin-like drugs found in oral contraceptives. Women who experience a hormonal menopause have been observed to experience the last menstrual bleed at a later age than women who experience menopause naturally, for example, 52.3 years versus 50.7 years (Treloar).

Artificial menopause is the induction of menopause by surgical removal of both ovaries and uterus (panhysterectomy: bilateral salpingectomy and oophorohysterectomy), or by ablative chemotherapy (through drugs such as Tamoxifen), or by radiation. Women who experience an artificial menopause have had menopause induced precipitously. The highest percentage of artificial menopause is surgically induced. Not long ago, about fifty percent of American women had undergone hysterectomy by age sixty (National Center for Health Statistics). A recent review article on women's health estimated the hysterectomy rate in the United States in the late 1980s at 1700 per day (Rodin and Ickovic). The occurrence of removal of ovaries in these cases has not been reported. Unfortunately, however, removal of healthy ovaries when a hysterectomy is performed is now recommended for all women over age forty (Sightler et al.). Whether ovaries are removed seems to depend on whether a woman's physician is a gynecologist or an endocrinologist (Stumpf).

Most endocrinologists recommend retaining the ovaries unless they are abnormal. These physicians believe that the ovaries are endocrine glands and, as such, are important sources of sex hormones for most postmenopausal women. The ovaries of most women develop a compensatory mechanism of estrogen synthesis involving certain cells that now have been identified as precursor cells of androgens, one of which, androstenedione, is converted to estrone in adipose (fatty) tissue. As much as thirty to fifty percent of this estrone precursor can be synthesized in a woman's ovaries postmenopausally (Utian 1987).

On the other hand, some gynecological oncologists, whether or not they believe that the postmenopausal ovary has no function, recommend ovary removal at hysterectomy. The rationale for performing ovary removal is based on an unsubstantiated belief that ovaries that are retained are at high risk for cancer, even though risk estimates of cancer in retained ovaries range from one in five hundred to one in five thousand women (Sightler et al.; Utian, in Lobo).

Common Changes

During the process of closure, somatic and affective changes occur. However, unlike the changes women reported during the premenstrual phase of the menstrual cycle (which are related to the sex steroids maximizing their mode of action in target tissue), as menopause approaches, certain changes indicate tissue response to the withdrawal of steroid hormones. Similar to premenstrual changes, these premenopausal changes are normal and predictable. They are a normal response to the withdrawal of estrogen, a substance that has been present in the body for more than thirty years. Some of the most common changes are hot flashes/flushes, heavy bleeding with clots, vaginal dryness, stress or urge incontinence, and mood swings.

Hot Flash/Flush. The medical term for "hot flash" is "vasomotor instability." A nontechnical, woman-generated definition of the phenomenon is "a perception of intense heat located in a specific body part." The hot flash may be best described as an emergency heat release mechanism. For reasons still unknown, as estrogen levels decrease, the fine tuning of the temperature-regulating mechanism in the brain and/or peripheral blood vessels is altered. Blood vessels that normally would open and close (dilate, constrict) when presented with an appropriate internal or external stimulus, such as increase or decrease in body heat, no longer fine tune. The hot flash is the most prevalent menopausal change; one study reported a prevalence rate of approximately eighty-nine percent (Feldman et al.).

Hot flashes may begin well in advance of the last menstrual bleed and may persist well beyond it (Voda 1981b). Information provided in the press and popular magazines claim that hot flashes will occur for a year or two, then subside. The temporal parameters of the experience have yet to be determined (Voda and George). For some women, the number of years of experiencing hot flashes both premenopausally and postmenopausally ranges from five to twenty (Voda 1981b). The highest frequency, intensity, and longest duration of hot flashes, however, occur around the time of menopause. Women can cope with the experience without hormones (Voda 1981b).

Vaginal and Urinary Changes. Some women experience vaginal dryness; thus, sexual activity may be painful if a woman is partnered with a male and if sexual activity is sporadic rather than regular. Cutler and Garcia recommend regular sexual activity, in other words, not feast or famine, as a way to maintain vaginal lubrication. If this is not possible, then a local application of creams, and in some cases estrogen hormone cream, will alleviate the dryness and prevent cracking and bleeding of tissue, which may provide a portal for micro-organisms and infection.

Burning and painful urination, as well as stress or urge incontinence, are not uncommon. Stress incontinence is the inability to retain urine when coughing, sneezing, running, and so on. Urge incontinence is the leaking of small quantities of urine prior to the active act of urinating. Voda (1984) found that seventy-five percent of menopausal women experienced either stress or urge incontinence which was unrelated to childbirth or bladder pathology. For many years women who complained of urinary incontinence were routinely treated with surgery in an attempt to suspend the bladder. Kegel exercises, traditionally taught to women after birthing or when urinary incontinence had become a problem, are a very effective noninvasive way of controlling incontinence. These exercises do not cure incontinence and are not the answer for uncontrollable symptoms (continual leakage). They do tone the perineal muscles and provide more control of urine retention. In recent years, two organizations have been founded to assist individuals with uncontrollable incontinence, HIP, Inc. (in Union, South Carolina), and The Simon Foundation (in Wilmette, Illinois).

Because the urethra is genitourinary tissue, it is estrogen-dependent tissue. True estrogen deficiency as a result of panhysterectomy will produce some urinary changes.

Mood Changes. Some women experience shifts in emotions around menopause. Brain cells also have receptors for estrogen. For the most part, these changes are not usually severe, and they are to be expected. Feminist research on this topic seems to suggest that mood swings are not totally due to hormone fluctuations. Rather, they may be more a result of physical changes (such as sleep loss due to hot flashes) or psychosocial changes occurring during the transitional period (Voda 1981b). In the premenopausal and postmenopausal years, women are faced with the reality of growing older in a culture that values youth. In addition, stress is increased at this time of life by children's postponing departure from the home, responsibility for aging parents, divorce, deaths, illness, and even suicide of family members (Voda and Mansfield in progress).

Bleeding Changes. Perhaps the most common change associated with the transition to menopause is the change in bleeding pattern. Not only does the bleeding interval change as menopause becomes imminent (Tre-

loar et al.), but changes in the quality and quantity of th
also occur. No data are available which describe how the
ing, for example, menstrual blood loss, changes. Work
(Voda and Mansfield in progress) suggests that the clos
menopause, the greater the possibility that her bleeding
clots for one to two days of a seven-day bleed. For a small number of
women the bleeding and clotting continue over a long period of time, for
example, fourteen days. This kind of bleeding pattern is not normal. However, because little or no normative data is available on how the bleeding
pattern changes premenopausally, any report by women to care providers
of heavy bleeding, clot passing, or a change in the pattern of bleeding, is
transformed into a medical diagnosis of "dysfunctional uterine bleeding."
Once this diagnosis is made, therapeutic interventions to correct the abnormal bleeding, such as hormone replacement or hysterectomy, become
viable options. Uterine fibroid tumors, which are benign, are postulated as
one source of heavy bleeding. These tumors have been described as "estrogen dependent." Why they occur and why they grow is only now the
focus of investigation. As ovulation decreases postmenopausally, estrogen
synthesis occurs without the antagonistic effect of progesterone. Because
the tumors have been characterized as estrogen dependent, they may grow
considerably during the premenopausal years.

In most women with fibroid tumors, if a hysterectomy is not performed, these tumors will shrink as estrogen levels continue to fall with
the approach of menopause. However, heavy or gushing bleeding over a
long duration is not normal and is reason to obtain the consultation of a
health-care provider (Cutler; Voda and Mansfield in progress).

Diseases Claimed to Be Preventable
with Estrogen Replacement

Osteoporosis. If endometrial cancer is the best-defined risk associated
with extended estrogen replacement therapy (ERT), the prevention of osteoporosis is declared the best-defined benefit (Barrett-Connor 1987,
1989). Osteoporosis, by definition, is a disease. It is demineralization and
thinning of bone, in which bone tissue density is reduced, increasing the
likelihood of fracture (Peck et al.). The process in individuals at risk begins
in the mid-thirties, and it occurs in both men and women. Like any other
disease, a family history of osteoporosis is a risk factor, but not the only
one. Osteoporosis has been defined as a multifactorial disorder (Peck et

. In women, early menopause, whether natural or induced, increases the risk of the disease as do age, race, body morphology, habits, and lifestyle (Peck et al.).

Estimates of the prevalence of osteoporosis vary widely, from one in four women (Notelovitz and Ware) to more than half of all white women (Cutler). Osteoporosis has been described as a worldwide medical problem confronting health-care workers (Cutler). This declaration emanated from reports of 247,000 hip fractures in 1985, mostly in women. It was predicted from this data that eight percent of women who were then thirty-five years of age (in 1985) would experience a hip fracture in later life. In 1986 the total female population of the United States was estimated at 50,336,000 (Rix). Eight percent of these women, or approximately four million, based on the 1985 estimates, would be at risk for hip fracture as they age. Based on these data, Hall, Davis, and Baran described osteoporosis as the disease of American women and recommended ERT for all menopausal women to prevent fractures and subsequent disability.

Epidemiological studies have documented the beneficial effect of estrogen with respect to a decreased risk of fractures in women who are at risk for osteoporosis. Based on these studies, proponents of ERT concluded that functional delay of menopause through administering estrogen would substantially decrease the risk of hip fractures (Peck et al.). Even though other agents have been shown to prevent bone loss leading to fractures (e.g., sodium fluoride, calcitonin, and a metabolite of vitamin D), the Food and Drug Administration approved oral, short-acting estrogen (estrone) at 0.625 mg, for twenty-five to twenty-six days. However, in order to protect the uterus from developing cancer, a progestin (medroxyprogesterone acetate [MPA] or depoprovera) must be administered along with estrogen from days 12–15 through 25. Thus, ERT became transformed into hormone replacement therapy (HRT). HRT was to be initiated as soon after menopause as possible and to continue for at least five to fifteen years.

Most postmenopausal women, however, do not need estrogen replacement to prevent osteoporosis. According to Yen, estrogen replacement is unnecessary and even contraindicated for a significant number of postmenopausal women. The lack of valid and reliable predictive methods to identify who should receive some form of prophylactic therapy for osteoporosis currently poses a major dilemma. For those women who would benefit from estrogen, acceleration in bone loss would have occurred before definitive evidence of entry into the menopausal transition (Yen).

The linking of osteoporosis with menopause has given new meaning to the horrors of Wilson's living decay (1966). This message has been translated into fear and concern and even some hysteria in women's magazines. The result has been to continue to medicalize menopause rather than acknowledge it as a normal process. For example, Seligson states in *Lears* that " . . . relief of symptoms is but a minor benefit . . . compared with ERT's proven ability to protect against heart disease and osteoporosis . . . osteoporosis is one of the true tragedies to befall women."

Sheehy perpetuates the doom and gloom in *Vanity Fair,* citing questionable statistics that one-third to one-half of all postmenopausal women and nearly half of all people over age seventy-five will be affected by this disease. While it is true that osteoporosis is a disease, it is, as I indicated earlier, a multifactorial disorder (Peck et al.). Clearly, for women who have a family history of osteoporosis, heredity is a risk factor. But so are age, race, and body build. Sheehy provides some hope for the baby boomers, whom she describes as bouncing from work to gym in nitrogen-cushioned aerobic shoes, popping calcium and snacking on veggies and yogurt. She contrasts these women with the elderly "frail" women who are now immobilized in nursing homes, implying that these women are stricken with osteoporosis because their formative years were calcium deficient and physically inactive. Perhaps there have been women born with silver spoons in their mouths, who then spent their lives sitting idly in parlors, one cross-stitching while another lazes at the piano, until they both tire and go to the garden for tea and canasta. Perhaps a few; but most of our mothers, grandmothers, and great-grandmothers were hard scrabble, hard working, physically active women who grew up in the heyday of milk and cheese, when food was real and fast food was a wary chicken. Sheehy has far too limited a perspective on the sociohistorical dynamics of both menopause and osteoporosis, and it leads her to false conclusions.

To Sheehy's credit, she forcefully notes that the politics surrounding osteoporosis are scandalous and that most medical plans do not reimburse for osteoporosis screening, nor is there a national screening program established or endorsed to diagnose early changes consistent with osteoporosis, as there is for breast cancer. As such, the words of Hall, Davis, and Baran continue to resonate throughout medical circles, linking menopause with osteoporosis and recommending estrogen replacement for all women even though only a small number of women are at risk for the disease (Yen).

Heart Disease. Whether estrogen replacement could prevent heart attacks in pre- and postmenopausal women was not a topic for medical debate until the 1980s (Barrett-Connor 1987). Past research on the risks related to oral contraceptive use suggested that the most serious risks to women were those related to the cardiovascular system; for example, heart attacks and strokes occurred more often in women who used the drugs than in women who did not (Hatcher et al.). In addition, results of an early study on men with heart disease reported higher levels of estrogen (estradiol) in heart-attack victims (Phillips et al.). Two studies in the 1970s on estrogen use in menopausal women reported an elevated risk of heart disease (Jick, Dinan, and Rothman; Jick, Dinan, Herman, and Rothman).

The 1980s brought a turning point in thinking about the potential risk/benefit ratio of estrogen in relation to heart disease when two studies reported a decreased risk of heart disease in women taking estrogen (Ross et al.; Bush et al.). Studies to determine whether estrogen replacement prevents heart disease in women became a top priority. In 1985 Stampfer et al., using data from a longitudinal survey, *The Nurses' Health Study,* concluded that estrogen use reduced the risk of severe coronary disease. Another report, based on data from the *Framingham Longitudinal Study,* concluded that no benefits from estrogen replacement were observed in women users; for example, mortality from all causes, including cardiovascular disease, did not differ among those who took estrogen and those who did not. An important finding from this report, which is not generally cited, was an increase in vascular disease in estrogen users (Wilson et al. 1985).

The next report to emanate from *The Nurses' Health Study* suggested that women who experienced natural menopause, having never used estrogen replacement, did not have an appreciable increase in the risk of coronary-artery disease when compared with premenopausal women. Women who were at risk were described as those who had bilateral oophorectomy and had never taken estrogen (Colditz et al.).

Using changes in lipoprotein levels as the indicators of risk for heart disease in estrogen users, Matthews et al. found an increase in low-density lipoprotein cholesterol and a decrease in high-density lipoprotein cholesterol. Data analyses were based on a comparison of sixty-nine naturally menopausal women who had had no period for twelve months and thirty-two women who had stopped menstruating on an average of six months and were on hormone replacement. The methodology of this study is somewhat problematic and is illustrative of the problems in much of the estrogen/heart disease prospective research designs. In this study, the differential effects of estrogen replacement from progesterone replacement and/or combination therapy (estrogen and progesterone) were not taken into account. The thirty-two women on hormone replacement were using all three kinds of hormone replacement. Additionally, while all sixty-nine menopausal women provided blood for follicle stimulating hormone (FSH) analyses and were declared menopausal based on FSH levels of more than thirty international units per liter, only twenty-four of the thirty-two women hormone users provided blood samples for FSH analyses. And of these twenty-four, only nineteen were defined as menopausal.

The most recent report from *The Nurses' Health Study* suggests that of the nurses who used estrogens, there was a fifty percent reduction in the incidence of coronary-artery disease (Stampfer et al. 1991). When data from this study were examined (to include the nurses who had been excluded because of cancer, preexisting heart disease, obesity, diabetes, etc.), the risk reduction for total mortality, not just deaths from heart disease, was insignificant (Wolfe; Vandenbroucke). In other words, the study findings suggest that women who elect to take hormones are probably healthier than women who do not take ERT or HRT.

Prior also has criticized *The Nurses' Health Study* as being biased in design and methodology, since the study was neither blinded or randomized. Prior has also objected that only risks for healthy women were reported. Including women with preexisting diseases and information on whether these women took estrogen, then stopped, because of migraines, swelling, or high blood pressure, would contribute important information about blood vessels, which might indicate that exogenous estrogens increase rather than decrease the risk for heart attack and other vascular problems (Wilson et al. 1985).

Fewer than twenty percent of American women at menopause are on hormone replacement therapy. The average length of time these women are on replacement hormones is nine months, and an estimated one-third of those who start out with HRT drop the progestin in about one year (Sheehy).

Another study of healthy women who used estrogen reported favorable alterations in healthy postmenopausal women's low- and high-density lipoprotein cholesterol levels (Walsh et al.). Also reported were increases in levels of plasma triglycerides; for example, in healthy women estrogen users with doses of 0.625 mg and 1.25 mg of Premarin, the triglycerides increased twenty-four percent and thirty-eight percent respectively. The researchers concluded that an increase of twenty-four percent involves no risk of inducing clinical hypertriglyceridemia (increased levels of blood lipids), which means an increase of twenty-four percent overall in circulating triglycerides in persons with normal levels. The researchers cautioned that in individuals with preexisting hypertriglyceridemia, estrogens should be used with caution. But this study, similar to the *Nurses' Health Study*, was biased. In addition, the validity of using indirect indicators, that is, levels of lipoprotein cholesterol, to support the assumption of an increased risk for heart disease in postmenopausal women is questionable. No data are presently available to document how lipid metabolism changes from pre- to postmenopause or whether changes that do occur place women at risk for heart disease.

The argument in support of estrogen use to prevent heart disease is based on the assumption that estrogen exerts a protective effect on cholesterol metabolism (Barrett-Connor 1987). Heart disease, like osteoporosis, is a multifactorial disease. In premenopausal women with cholesterol levels higher than 240 mg/deciliter, heart disease is rare unless other risk factors (high blood pressure, obesity, smoking, high alcohol consumption, diabetes, or preexisting heart disease, such as familial hypercholesterolemia) are present. Proponents of estrogen therapy imply that these particular risks in men and women even out after women reach menopause.

Just how estrogen prevents heart attacks in women is unknown. Evidence to date is either epidemiological or indirect. The indirect evidence, as I have mentioned, is based on changes in the lipid profile—lipoprotein cholesterol and triglyceride levels (Matthews et al.; Walsh et al.), factors that have been identified as either high- or low-risk factors from studies on men. In addition, eliminating from these and other studies women who were smokers, obese, diabetic, hypertensive, who had abnormal blood lipids, or who consumed more than 28 ml of ethanol per day, limits study findings. In the Walsh et al. study, in particular, a progestin, MPA, was given to study participants who used estrone ten days after completion of the study to remove any hyperplastic endometrium. Study findings, therefore, are limited to the effects of estrone alone, given by mouth to healthy women who had uteruses. However, in the long run, study findings are academic, since a healthy postmenopausal woman who has not undergone hysterectomy must take estrogen with a progestin to protect her uterus from becoming hyperplastic (Schenken and Pauerstein). Progestins commonly used with ERT are norethindrone, Norgestrel, and oral progesterone. Combining a progestin with estrogen (even the less potent MPA) for the required twelve days each month has raised substantial concern that the beneficial effects on cardiac disease, mediated via changes in serum lipid profiles, may be eliminated (Schenken and Pauerstein; Lobo; Notelovitz; Utian 1990).

Breast Cancer. Evidence suggesting that estrogen use, via oral contraceptives or ERT at menopause, increases the risk of breast cancer is a continuing source of concern. Until the Bergkvist et al. study on Swedish women and estrogen use was reported, no definitive evidence that ERT increased the risk of breast cancer was available. As mentioned earlier, many investigations failed to demonstrate an increased risk of breast cancer in oral-contraceptive users (Hatcher et al.). Only one study (Pike et al.) postulated an increased risk of breast cancer in young women using oral contraceptives with a high progestin component. Based upon the finding of low risk for oral-contraceptive users, and one large study supporting the protective effects of hormone replacement therapy on the breast (Gambrel et al.), combination HRT was recommended for women with or without a uterus in order to protect them from developing breast cancer (Barrett-Connor 1987).

Results of the Bergkvist et al. study have now changed the way clinicians think about postmenopausal HRT (Barrett-Connor 1989). Bergkvist et al. reported that Swedish women who had used estrogen alone (in the form of estradiol) as ERT for at least nine years carried nearly double the risk of breast cancer. Critics of the study were quick to note that estradiol is not the estrogen taken by women in the United States. Rather, women in the United States take estrone, E_1. The critics, however, have not said why estrone would not present as much risk as estradiol, since both steroids would bind with cytosolic and nuclear estrogen receptors to promote the desired protective effect.

According to Barrett-Connor (1989), a most provocative finding of the Bergkvist et al. study was a four-fold increase in the risk of breast cancer in women who used combination therapy (estrogen plus a progestin). Although this association was not statistically supported, it was similar to the findings of another study (Pike et al.), which was followed up with a hypothesis that estrogen and progestin combinations are more carcinogenic to women than estrogens alone (Key and Pike).

A review of all the epidemiological studies on the effect of ERT on the risk of breast cancer, reported as a meta-analysis, suggested that the longer a woman uses estrogen, the greater the risk of cancer (Steinberg et al.). The strength of this study was in its methodology. It controlled for the quality of the reported research using specific criteria. Of those studies that were evaluated as "high" in quality, five reported an increased risk for breast cancer, whereas those studies that were evaluated as "low" in quality reported no increased risk for breast cancer (Steinberg et al.). The findings of the meta-analysis were incorporated into the *Federal Register* through testimony given by Sidney Wolfe to the Senate Subcommittee on Aging in April of 1991 (Wolfe).

Finally, the work of Russo and Russo and their hypotheses regarding breast cancer and hormones as carcinogens have not been given sufficient attention. These investigators believe that breast cancer arises from undifferentiated breast structures, defined as terminal ducts. Normally, breast tissue development is directed by endogenous estrogen and progesterone. During pregnancy particularly, or during ovulatory menstrual cycles, estrogen directs breast ductal development (i.e., cells proliferate and increase in number). The result of cellular proliferation is the formation of breast tissue structures referred to as "terminal end buds" or TEBs. In the presence of progesterone, these TEBs differentiate into structures called alveolar buds (ABs). The researchers observed that in rats the terminal end buds that did not differentiate into alveolar buds atrophied. These shrunken TEBs are referred to as "terminal ducts." Russo and Russo have hypothesized that adding progestins to estrogen in HRT has the potential to increase the risk of breast cancer by activating the atrophied terminal ducts.

Another hypothesis advanced by Russo and Russo relates to the timing of hormone influence in the process of breast development. On manipulating hormones in rats, they found that the earlier pregnancy occurred in the life of a mature animal, the greater the protection against cancer from the effect of progesterone in differentiating (transforming) terminal end buds into alveolar buds and lobules. They hypothesized that a similar effect might be derived from lower levels of progesterone synthesized during ovulatory menstrual cycles (in the case of the rat, during estrous cycles). This hypothesis has particular implications for young postmenarchal women engaged in long-term (ten to fifteen years) use of hormonal contraceptives. The desired action of hormonal contraceptives is stopping ovulation to prevent pregnancy. If ovulation is prevented, endogenous progesterone synthesis does not occur. Whether differentiation of breast tissue occurs with exogenous progesterone found in hormonal contraceptives is unknown.

Hence, another dilemma related to hormone use has arisen. Young postmenarchal women are considered high risk for pregnancy. The recommendation regarding contraception is to prescribe hormonal contraceptives to young women as soon as possible after sexual maturation (Hatcher et al.). If these women remain on hormonal contraceptives for a long period of time, even in low doses, and the contraceptives effectively prevent ovulation, the normal process of breast tissue differentiation normally mediated via endogenous hormones will be altered.

Finally, related to hormone replacement for postmenopausal women, Russo and Russo have hypothesized that if tissue is stimulated through HRT (both estrogen and progesterone), both TEBs and ABs are at risk of cancerous transformation, since stimulation of these structures is occurring out of the protective window, that is ages twelve to twenty-four, when maximal hormone stimulation normally occurs to promote development of breast tissue.

Conclusion

On average, women who live in westernized cultures can expect to live more than thirty years past menopause. As the construction of menopause as disease or endocrinopathy continues to dominate thinking about menopause, healthy midlife women are increasingly encouraged to replace hormones. If they live long enough, all women, one way or another, experience menopause, and will experience some degree of decline in estrogen levels from levels occurring during their prime reproductive years. However, most postmenopausal women will not experience serious illnesses or diseases as a result of not receiving supplemental or additive estrogens (Notelovitz; Utian 1987).

Estrogen may not only be appropriate but essential for women with certain pathological states, for example, those who have had menopause induced prematurely via surgery, radiation, or chemotherapy (Notelovitz). In these women, estrogen replacement to prevent osteoporosis, if risk factors for this disease are present, may be appropriate, since early menopause shortens the time during which natural estrogens are synthesized in the body. For most women, however, the transit to menopause is gradual and they are not estrogen deficient. Rather, they have been made estrogen deficient when hysterectomy has been performed and perfectly healthy ovaries have been removed. Removal of a woman's ovaries is castration. Removal of healthy ovaries in a healthy pre- or postmenopausal woman is unnecessary and might well be considered malpractice, since the ovary is an endocrine gland which has a function continuing into postmenopausal life.

Normally, androgens synthesized in a postmenopausal woman's ovary diffuse into the circulation. When they reach the adipose tissue, they are converted into estrone (E_1) through an enzymatic process referred to as aromatization. In this process, an androgenic steroid, androstenedione (A), is converted to estrone. The estrone synthesized in the fatty tissue diffuses into the circulation and is available to interact with receptors inside target cells. That there is such a process and that it becomes more efficient with age has been known since the early 1970s (Grodin et al.). This process is undoubtedly one reason for the variability of experiences in menopause among women, that is, the number of changes experienced, as well as the frequency and intensity of complaints related to estrogen withdrawal from cells.

Even though estrone is weaker than estradiol, the dominant hormone during reproductive years, it binds with target cell receptors to induce estrogen receptor mediated events. If estrone were not effective, estrogen replacement in the form of estrone, as found in Premarin, would not be prescribed for women.

Hysterectomy with precipitous, iatrogenic castration induces menopause and estrogen deficiency. The younger a woman is when she has been castrated, the longer she can expect to be on ERT and, consequently, the greater the risks to health. Whether a woman takes ERT or HRT because she has been made estrogen deficient or because she has been made to believe that she is estrogen deficient, she needs to understand that hormones alter metabolic processes in a variety of ways that are known to be risky. And the unknown risks may meet or surpass the known risks. When menopausal symptoms, such as hot flashes, diminish or subside with hormone use, the woman clearly has experienced a positive, desired effect of the hormone interacting with receptors in certain tissues. In the uterus, however, estrogens produce an indiscernible, undesirable effect. If a progestin is not administered with the estrogen, uterine cells will proliferate in an unregulated manner. The sequelae of cell proliferation may result in cancer (Schenken and Pauerstein). To regulate and control the unwanted and uncontrolled effect of estrogen-mediated cell division, medical researchers advocate prescribing estrogen with a progestin. Adding a progestin is an attempt to mimic events that occur in the menstrual cycle during a woman's prime reproductive years. The rub here is that the menstrual cycle was genetically preprogrammed for closure at around age fifty, and there is almost no research available showing that either estrogen or progestin administration to women over the long term is safe generally or protective of the uterus. For example, few studies have been done which document combining various progestins with estrogen to effect the prevention of endometrial disease. Although the metabolic pathways of the commonly prescribed progestins are well described, little data is available on the biological activity of the metabolites, that is, what happens once the progestin enters the system or after it binds with the uterine receptor. This, as well as the variable rates of metabolism in women, is an important and unknown factor that may influence how the various compounds affect the endometrium (Schenken and Pauerstein). If these compounds are found to have a negative effect on the endometrium, the result may be an increase in the hysterectomy rate, which is estimated at more than 1700 a day, as I mentioned earlier (Rodin and Ickovic).

Related to breast cancer, the findings of Bergkvist et al. and Steinberg et al. link estrogen with an increased risk of breast cancer, which is cause for immediate concern for women's health. In a few short years, the incidence of breast cancer in the United States has increased from one in fourteen to one in nine. The risks associated with the addition of a progestin are unknown. However, Bergkvist et al. suggested that there was an increased risk for breast cancer in Swedish women who used combined therapy.

With all of the unknowns related to hormone therapy for women and all of the risks that have been identified in users, it is instructive at this point to recall the concerns raised by Hellman about healthy people taking powerful drugs for a purpose other than to prevent or treat a disease. Since Hellman's message to physicians, much has been learned about the mechanism of action of steroids in general. We know that the sex steroids in target tissue induce two main functions via a receptor-mediated process: they induce protein synthesis, for example, synthesis of enzymes and growth factors, and in the uterus and breast they promote cell division. The final intracellular receptor for all steroids lies within the nucleus, on the genome, the spiral strand of DNA.

If we consider the heritage of the genes, we learn that many messages have been there for ages. Some messages function to mature the woman, some promote conception, some sustain pregnancy; others bring a timely closure to processes, like menstrual life. For almost a quarter of a century, well women have been manipulating and altering the function of their DNA with steroidal hormones, first with birth-control pills, then with estrogen replacement, and now with combination hormone replacement. An indisputable result of this manipulation has been a prescription for hazard and even death for some women. Among the known consequences of hormone use are genitourinary cancers for young women and men whose mothers used DES in the 1940s and 1950s to prevent miscarriage (Herbst et al.); strokes and heart attacks in women who used the pill in the 1960s and 1970s (Seaman and Seaman; Voda 1981a); uterine cancer from estrogen replacement in the 1970s (Smith et al.; Ziel and Finkle; Mack et al.); breast cancer for women who took DES in the 1960s (Greenberg et al.) and for women who accepted hormone replacement in the 1980s (Bergkvist et al.; Steinberg et al.).

Survival of the human species has always depended upon the ability of body cells during the reproductive years to express gene-hormone messages appropriately. Disease-free survival and postmenopausal life quality may depend on the ability of women and their care providers to heed the message from the center of the cells, the genome; that is, there is a time to manipulate genes with endogenous hormones in a natural and regulated way, as during the menstrual or pregnancy cycle (Russo and Russo), and there is a time to bring closure to the process, not prolong it with exogenous hormone replacement at menopause or alter it during reproductive life with steroidal contraceptives to prevent pregnancy.

Women who elect to take hormones for birth control, perhaps for a long period of time, starting at an early postmenarchal age, have in effect turned off normal processes that regulate growth and development of the reproductive system and perhaps other processes as yet unknown. Particularly worrisome is the role that these hormones may play in causing breast cancer, since with the suppression of ovulation caused by steroidal contraceptives, breast tissue cannot maximally differentiate. As mentioned, whether these undifferentiated structures will be more susceptible to carcinogens or hormonal transformation is unknown. And the population in whom and on whom we are awaiting the results are healthy women who have been urged to take steroid hormones, having been convinced that taking them is safe.

Health-care providers try to help sick people move toward health. Health-care providers also try to help well people stay well. Health-care providers do not generally in good conscience dispense drugs or condone devices that interrupt or alter normal physiological processes in well people, thereby producing illness. As a health-care provider, I have been concerned about hormone use for a long time because I know that the hormones have many side effects, and I understand how these side effects are produced. As a nurse, a woman, and a feminist, I am concerned that these effects have been and will continue to be experienced by healthy women. Which women these will be we do not know and we cannot predict.

Advocates for hormone use, whether for birth control or for hormone replacement, insist that the benefits of use outweigh the risks. For example, those who advocate steroidal contraceptives argue that death from complications associated with pregnancy are far greater than the risks associated with using steroidal contraceptives (pitting one normal process in women against another). For estrogen or hormone replacement therapy, the benefits of preventing osteoporosis and heart disease are held to outweigh the risks related to any cancer that will be caused—pitting disease against disease: which one would you choose?

In 1981 I questioned the criteria used in deriving the risk/benefit equation for oral contraceptive use. The criteria employed were the same as those used when assessing risk in treating disease. For example, when considering a new treatment for a person who is sick, that treatment is weighed against the risks and benefits of the other options open to the person. For the cancer patient, then, the benefit of drug taking is presumed to outweigh the risks associated with its sometimes toxic and iatrogenic side effects as compared to no treatment or a conventional treatment. The benefit of drug treatment in a case like this, that is, the chance to live, far outweighs the risk. But the situation is just not this clear when we attempt a risk/benefit analysis in the case of hormone use, because we are dealing with healthy people (Voda 1981a).

The World Health Organization definition of health asserts that everyone has a fundamental right to the highest attainable standard of health without distinction based on race, religion, politics, or socioeconomic status (Beauchamp and Walters). This definition needs to modified to include gender. It is highly questionable that women who take steroidal contraceptives or hormone replacement therapy enjoy or will achieve the highest attainable standard of health, since these women are put at risk of chronic disease resulting from the use of these hormones. Do women have less of a right to health than men, who face no pressure to take exogenous hormones through the whole of their adult lives?

Wolfe has also raised this issue. Regarding the risks of breast cancer associated with hormone use, he observes: If a drug which had the potential to reduce heart disease in men were available and considered for national use but was known to cause testicular cancer, doctors would refuse to prescribe it and their patients would refuse to use it (Wolfe).

In Houston, Texas a male sex offender pleaded with his judge to be castrated to stop him from offending again. Castration (removal of the testicles) would take the place of a long prison sentence. The judge agreed with the man's request but had to reconsider the prison sentence when no doctor could be found to perform the surgery (Associated Press).

In contrast, gynecological surgeons have no difficulty deciding whether or not to castrate women. As I have already twice mentioned, it is currently estimated that 1,700 hysterectomies are performed every day in the United States. Of these, approximately thirty percent include female castration (National Center for Health Statistics), because practice standards established by gynecological surgeons recommend removal of the ovaries when hysterectomy is done in order to prevent ovarian cancer. For some castrated women to have even a semblance of quality life, the only option is hormone replacement.

Every year 320,000 American men, most over 60, undergo surgery for benign enlargement of the prostate. Since 1989, men in the Denver-based Kaiser Permanente Health Plan who have prostate enlargement have been required to view (as part of an attempt to reduce health-care costs) a forty-five-minute video which explains in plain, unbiased terms the risks and benefits of the surgery. The result of this educational intervention has been a forty-five percent reduction in the number of prostate surgeries performed (Faltermeyer). Men have just said no, and for good reason.

Hysterectomies in this country are usually performed to correct a benign or misdiagnosed condition, such as dysfunctional uterine bleeding, whether this is caused by fibroids (benign tumors) or is simply a normal change in the menstrual bleeding pattern. Since physicians do not regard a woman's uterus as an important organ once reproductive life has ended, treatment for fibroids and/or dysfunctional bleeding has been to remove the organ surgically (Cutler). Research indicates that women experience a variety of affective and somatic changes following "simple" hysterectomy, that is, hysterectomy not involving castration (Cutler).

A strategy similar to the one used with the men who were asked to view the videotape on prostate surgery, which clearly explains the risks, including the risks associated with ovary removal and subsequent hormone therapy, would end the hysterectomy epidemic in this country and draw attention to a long-standing unethical medical practice, removal of healthy ovaries from women's bodies.

Given our knowledge of how the sex hormones function in the human body and given the data presently available suggesting serious risks to women's health, using hormones to intervene in a natural process is unhealthy and unethical. The ever-present controversy over the risks and potential benefits of hormone use has been illogically conceived, since risk/benefit criteria for drug use in healthy people is not the same as it is for sick people. That well-intentioned but ill-informed mythologies persist about women and events associated with menstruation, reproduction, and menopause is an understatement. They thrive at the very highest bureaucratic levels of health care. In spite of all that we know, a multisite research project, the "postmenopausal estrogen/progestin interventions trial" (PEPI), has been funded by the National Institutes of Health to determine what combinations of female hormones will be the most beneficial for postmenopausal women. The entire framework of this research is based on the model of menstruation, reproduction, and menopause as diseases rather than as natural events. The theoretical framework in which this research is grounded is Wilson's ideology of women as estrogen deficient at menopause. Research undertaken in this framework does not seek answers to how women can most healthily live their lives; rather it seeks to cure women of being women. If we have come full circle back to the mythmakers of yesteryear, it is because we have never departed from the age-old fears, hostilities, and superstitions connected to women's reproductive capacities. It is time to do better.

REFERENCES

American Cancer Society Breast Cancer Task Force (1991). *Facts about breast cancer in the USA.* American Cancer Society, Larchmont, N.Y.

Asso, D. (1983). *The real menstrual cycle.* John Wiley & Sons, New York.

Associated Press (1992). Surgeons say no, so rape suspect won't be castrated. *Salt Lake Tribune,* 17 March, 1992.

Barrett-Connor, E. (1987). Postmenopausal estrogen, cancer and other considerations. *Women and Health* 32:179–95.

———. (1989). Postmenopausal estrogen replacement and breast cancer. *New England Journal of Medicine* 321:319–20.

Beauchamp, T. L., and Walters, L. (1978). *Contemporary issues in bioethics.* Dickensen, Belmont, Calif.

Beral, V. (1976). Cardiovascular-disease mortality trends and oral contraceptive use in young women. *Lancet* 2:1047–52.

———. (1977). Mortality among oral contraceptive users. *Lancet* 2:727–31.

Bergkvist, L.; Adami, H.; Persson, I.; Hoover, R.; and Schairer, C. (1989). The risk of breast cancer after estrogen and estrogen-progestin replacement. *New England Journal of Medicine* 321 (5):293–97.

Bloch, E. (1953). Quantitative morphological investigations of the follicular system in newborn female infants. *Acta Anatomy* 17:201.

Bush, T. L.; Cowan, L. D.; Barrett-Connor, E.; et al. (1983). Estrogen use and all cause mortality: Preliminary results from the Lipid Research Clinics Program Follow-Up Study. *JAMA* 249:903–906.

Colditz, C. A.; Willett, W. C.,; Stampfer, M. J.; Rosner, B.; Speizer, F. E.; and Hennekens, C. H. (1987). Menopause and risk of coronary heart disease in women. *New England Journal of Medicine* 316:1105–10.

Cutler, W. B. (1988). *Hysterectomy before and after.* Harper and Row, New York.

Cutler, W. B., and Garcia, R. (1992). *Menopause: A guide for women and the men who love them.* Norton, New York.

Dan, A.; Graham, E. A.; and Beecher, C. P. (eds.) (1980). *The menstrual cycle. Vol. I: A synthesis of interdisciplinary research.* Springer, New York.

Delaney, J.; Lupton, J. J.; and Toth, E. (1988). *The curse: A cultural history of menstruation.* University of Illinois Press, Urbana.

Faltermayer, E. (1992). Let's really cure the health care system. *Fortune,* 46–58.

Fausto-Sterling, A. (1985). *Myths of gender.* Basic Books, New York.

Feldman, B. M.; Voda, A. M.; and Gronseth, E. (1985). Prevalence of hot flash and associated variables in perimenopausal women. *Research in Nursing and Health* 8:261–68.

Frank, R. T. (1931). The hormonal causes of premenstrual syndrome. *Archives of Neurology and Psychiatry* 26:1053.

Gambrel, R., Jr.; Maier, R.; and Sanders, B. (1983). Decreased incidence of breast cancer in postmenopausal estrogen-progesten users. *Obstetrics and Gynecology* 62:435–43.

Golub, S. (ed.) (1983). *Lifting the curse of menstruation.* Haworth, New York.

Goodman, M. (1991). Menopause research 1979–1989. In *Proceedings of the 8th conference society for menstrual cycle research.* A. M. Voda and R. Conover (eds.). Society for Menstrual Cycle Research, Salt Lake City. 141–60.

Greenberg, E. R.; Barnes, A. B.; Resseguie, L.; Barrett, J. A.; Burnside, S.; Lauza, L. L.; Neff, R. K.; Stevens, M.; Young, R. H.; and Colton, T. (1984). Breast cancer in mothers given diethylstilbesterol in pregnancy. *New England Journal of Medicine* 311:1393–98.

Grodin, M.; Siiteri, P. K.; and MacDonald, P. C. (1973). Source of estrogen production in postmenopausal women. *Journal of Clinical Endocrinology and Metabolism* 36:207–14.

Hall, F. M.; Davis, M. A.; and Baran, D. T. (1987). Bone mineral screening for osteoporosis. *New England Journal of Medicine* 316:212–14.

Hatcher, R. A.; Stewart, F.; Trussell, J.; Kowal, D.; Guest, F.; Stewart, G. K.; and Cates, W. (1990). *Contraceptive technology 1990–1992.* Irvington, New York.

Hellman, I. M. (1975). Fertility control at a crossroad. *American Journal of Obstetrics and Gynecology* 124:331–37.

Herbst, A. L.; Robboy, S. J.; Scully, B. E.; et al. (1974). Clear cell adenoma of the vagina and cervix in girls: An analysis of 170 registry cases. *American Journal of Obstetrics* 119:713–24.

Jick, H.; Dinan, B.; Herman, R.; and Rothman, K. J. (1978). Myocardial infarction and other vascular diseases in young women: Role of estrogens and other factors. *JAMA* 240:2548–52.

Jick, H.; Dinan, B.; and Rothman, K. J. (1978). Noncontraceptive estrogens and nonfatal myocardial infarction. *JAMA* 239:1407–1408.

Key, T. J. A., and Pike, M. C. (1988). The role of oestrogens and progestogens in the epidemiology and prevention of breast cancer. *European Journal of Clinical Oncology* 24:29–43.

Keye, W. R. (1988). *The premenstrual syndrome.* W. B. Saunders, Philadelphia.

Kistner, R. W. (1969). *The pill. Facts and fallacies about today's oral contraceptives.* Dell, New York.

Komnenich, P.; McSweeney, M.; Noack, J. A.; and Elder, N. (eds.) (1981). *The menstrual cycle. Vol. II: Research and implications for women's health.* Springer, New York.

Korenman, S. G.; Sherman, B. M.; and Korenman, J. C. (1978). Reproductive hormone function: The perimenopausal period and beyond. *Clinics in Endocrinology and Metabolism* 7:625–43.

Lander, L. (1988). *Images of bleeding.* Orlando, New York.

Lobo, R. A. (1990). Cardiovascular implications of estrogen replacement therapy. *Obstetrics and Gynecology* 75:18s–35s.

Mack, T.; Pike, M.; Henderson, B.; Pfeffer, R.; Gerkins, V.; Authur, M.; and Braun, S. (1976). Estrogens and endometrial cancer in a retirement community. *New England Journal of Medicine* 294:1262–67.

MacPherson, K. I. (1981). Menopause as disease: The social construction of a metaphor. *Advances in Nursing Science* 3:95–113.

———. (1985). Osteoporosis and menopause: A feminist analysis of the social construction of a syndrome. *Advances in Nursing Science* 7:11–21.

———. (1991). Hormone replacement therapy for menopause: A contrast between medical and women's health movement perspectives. In *Proceedings of the 8th conference society for menstrual cycle research*. A. M. Voda and R. Conover (eds.). Society for Menstrual Cycle Research, Salt Lake City.

Martin, E. (1988). Medical metaphors of women's bodies: Menstruation and menopause. *International Journal of Health Services* 18:237–54.

Matthews, K. A.; Meilahn, E.; Kuller, L. H.; Kelsey, S. F.; Caggiula, A. W.; and Wing, R. R. (1989). Menopause and risk factors for coronary heart disease. *New England Journal of Medicine* 321:641–46.

National Center for Health Statistics (1987). DHHS Publication #(DHS)88-1753. USDHHS, PHS, CDC, December, Washington, D.C.

National Women's Health Network (1989). *Taking hormones and women's health: Choices, risks and benefits*. National Women's Health Network, Washington, D.C.

Notelovitz, M. (1989). An opposing view. *Journal of Family Practice* 29 (4): 410–15.

Notelovitz, M., and Ware, M. (1982). *Stand tall: the informed woman's guide to preventing osteoporosis*. Triad, Gainesville, Fla.

O'Malley, B. W., and Schrader, W. T. (1976). The receptors of steroid hormones. *Scientific American* 234:32–43.

Peck, W. A.; Riggs, B. L.; and Bell, N. H. (1987). *Physician's resource manual on osteoporosis: A decision-making guide*. National Osteoporosis Foundation, Washington, D.C.

Phillips, G. B.; Castelli, W. P.; Abbott, R. D.; and McNamara, P. M. (1983). Association of Hyperestrogenemia and coronary heart disease in men in the Framingham cohort. *American Journal of Medicine* 74:863–69.

Pike, M. C.; Henderson, B. E.; Krailo, M. D.; Duke, A.; and Roy, S. (1983). Breast cancer in young women and use of oral contraceptives: Possible modifying effect of formulation and age at use. *Lancet* 11:926–30.

Prior, J. C. (1992). Critique of estrogen treatment for heart attack prevention: The nurses health study. *A Friend Indeed* 7 (8):3–5.

Rix, S. E. (1990). *The American woman 1990–1991*. W. W. Norton, New York.

Rodin, J., and Ickovic, J. R. (1990). Women's health: Review and research agenda as we approach the 21st century. *American Psychologist* 45:1018–34.

Ross, R. K.; Paganini-Hill, A.; Mack, T. M.; Arthur, M.; and Henderson, B. E. (1981). Menopausal oestrogen therapy and protection from death and ischaemic heart disease. *Lancet* 1:858–60.

Russo, J., and Russo, I. H. (1987). Biological and molecular bases of mammary carcinogenesis. *Laboratory Investigation* 57:112–37.

Schenken, R. S., and Pauerstein, C. J. (1989). Effects of progestogens on the endometrium. In *Menopause: Evaluation, treatment, and health concerns*. C B. Hammond, F. I. Haseltine, and I. Schiff (eds.). Alan R. Liss, New York. 1–28.

Seaman, B., and Seaman, G. (1977). *Women and the crisis in sex hormones*. Rawson Associates, New York.

Seligson, M. (1990). Body briefing: Estrogen replacement. *Lears* 3:54–62.

Sheehy, G. (1991). The silent passage: Menopause. *Vanity Fair* 54:222–63.

Sightler, S. E.; Boike, G. M.; Estape, R. E.; and Averette, H. E. (1991). Ovarian cancer in women with prior hysterectomy: A 14-year experience at the University of Miami. *Obstetrics and Gynecology* 78:681.

Silverberg, E. (1984). Cancer statistics. *Cancer* 34:7–23.

Smith, D. C.; Prentice, R.; Thompson, D. J.; and Herrman, W. L. (1975). Association of exogenous estrogen and endometrial carcinoma among users of conjugated estrogens. *New England Journal of Medicine* 293:1167–70.

Stadel, B., and Weiss, N. (1975). Characteristics of menopausal women: A survey of King and Pierce counties in Washington, 1973–1974. *Journal of Epidemiology* 102:215.

Stampfer, M. J.; Colditz, G. A.; Willett, W. C.; Manson, J. A. E.; Rosner, B.; Speizer, F. E.; and Hennekens, C. H. (1991). Postmenopausal estrogen therapy and cardiovascular disease. *New England Journal of Medicine* 325:756–62.

Stampfer, M. J.; Willett, W. C.; Colditz, G. A.; Rosner, B.; Speizer, F. E.; and Hennekens, C. H. (1985). A prospective study of postmenopausal estrogen therapy and coronary heart disease. *New England Journal of Medicine* 313:1044–49.

Steinberg, K. K.; Thacker, S. B.; Smith, S. J.; Stroup, D. F.; Zack, M. M.; Flanders, W. D.; and Berkelman, L. R. (1991). A meta-analysis of the effect of estrogen replacement therapy on the risk of breast cancer. *JAMA* 265:1985–90.

Stumpf, J., in Lobo, R. A. (1990). Panel discussion 2: Cardiovascular implications of estrogen replacement therapy. *Obstetrics and Gynecology* 75:31s–35s.

Taylor, D. (1988). *The red flower: Rethinking menstruation.* Crossing, Freedom, Calif.

Treloar, A. E. (1981). Menstrual cyclicity and the pre-menopause. *Maturitas* 3:249–64.

Treloar, A. E.; Boynton, R. E.; Bohn, G. G.; and Brown, B. W. (1967). Variation of the human menstrual cycle through reproductive life. *International Journal of Fertility* 12:77–127.

Utian, W. H. (1987). Overview on menopause. *American Journal of Obstetrics and Gynecology* 156:1280–83.

———. (1990). The Menopause in perspective. *Multidisciplinary Perspectives on Menopause* 592:1–7. Annals of the New York Academy of Sciences, New York.

Utian, W. H., in Lobo, R. A. (1990). Cardiovascular implications of estrogen replacement therapy. *Obstetrics and Gynecology.* 75:18s–35s.

Vandenbrouke, J. P. (1991). Postmenopausal oestrogen and cardioprotection. *Lancet* 337:833–34.

Voda, A. M. (1980). Pattern of progesterone and aldosterone in ovulatory women during the menstrual cycle. In *The menstrual cycle. Vol. I: A synthesis of interdisciplinary research.* A. J. Dan, E. A. Graham, and C. P. Beecher (eds.). Springer, New York. 223–36.

———. (1981a). Alterations of the menstrual cycle: Hormonal and mechanical. In *The menstrual cycle. Vol. II.* P. Komnenich, M. E. McSweeney, J. A. Noak, and N. Elder (eds.). Springer, New York. 145–63.

———. (1981b). Climacteric hot flash. *Maturitas* 1:1–21.

———. (1984). *Final report research grant #R01NU00961,* unpublished report, USPHS Division of Nursing.

Voda, A. M.; Dinnerstein, M.; and O'Donnell, S. (eds.) (1982). *Changing perspectives on menopause.* University of Texas Press, Austin.

Voda, A. M., and Eliasson, M. (1983). Menopause: The closure of menstrual life.

In *Lifting the curse of menstruation*. S. Golub (ed.). Haworth, New York. 137–56.

Voda, A. M., and George, T. (1986). Menopause. In *Annual Review of Nursing Research 4*. H. H. Werley, J. J. Fitzpatrick, and R. L. Taunton (eds.). 55–75.

Voda, A. M., and Mansfield, P. K. (in progress). Menopause and midlife changes. Unpublished working paper.

———. (in press). Change in bleeding pattern in premenopausal women. In *Proceedings 9th conference society for menstrual cycle research*. N. Woods (ed.). University of Washington, Seattle.

Voda, A. M., and Randall, M. P. (1982). Nausea and vomiting of pregnancy: "Morning sickness." In *Concept clarification in nursing*. C. M. Norris (ed.). Aspen, Rockville, Md.

Walsh, B. W.; Schiff, I.; Rosner, B.; Greenberg, L.; Ravnikar, V.; and Sacks, F. M. (1991). Effects of postmenopausal estrogen replacement on the concentrations and metabolism of plasma lipoproteins. *New England Journal of Medicine* 325:1196–1204.

Wilson, P. W. F.; Garrison, R. J.; and Castelli, W. P. (1985). Postmenopausal estrogen use, cigarette smoking, and cardiovascular morbidity in women over 50. *New England Journal of Medicine* 313:1038–43.

Wilson, R. (1966). *Feminine forever*. M. Evans, New York.

Wilson, R., and Wilson, T. A. (1963). The fate of nontreated postmenopausal women: A plea for the maintenance of adequate estrogen from puberty to the grave. *Journal of the American Geriatric Society* 11:347–62.

Wolfe, S. M. (1992). Estrogen, breast cancer, heart disease. *A Friend Indeed* 7 (8):1–3.

Yen, S. S. C. (1986). Estrogen withdrawal syndrome. *New England Journal of Medicine* 255:1014.

Ziel, H. K., and Finkle, W. D. (1975). Increased risk of endometrial carcinoma among users of conjugated estrogens. *New England Journal of Medicine* 293:1167–70.

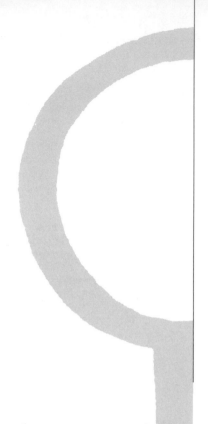

Medical Decision Making: Issues Concerning Menopause

Rosalind Ekman Ladd

The long and infamous tradition of parentalism in the medical care of women has been well documented (Notman and Nadelson; Ehrenreich and English). It would be neither novel nor radical to argue that grown women should not be treated like children and that all competent adults have a right to make decisions for themselves.

Beyond this, however, there are certain features of medical decision making in the context of menopause that are significantly different from decisions in other areas of health care and which constitute persuasive grounds, I think, for challenging the role of physicians as primary decision makers.

My purpose in this paper is to provide a careful analysis of the nature of medical decision making around issues of menopause, drawing out the implications for needed changes in the customary doctor/patient relationship.

Some may question the appropriateness of focusing on medical decision making for menopausal women. The feminist position is that menopause is part of the normal aging process and that issues about women's health care are and should be understood as social issues, not medical problems (McCrea). Nevertheless, physicians continue to define menopause as a deficiency disease, and some experts estimate that as many as seventy-five percent of all menopausal women have symptoms severe enough to lead them to seek medical consultation (Brenner).[1] Thus, the frequency of interaction between physicians and menopausal women and the tendency toward medicalization of menopause and related phenomena by physicians suggest that discussion of medical decision making in the context of menopause is needed.

Parentalism in the doctor/patient relationship is characterized by the physician making decisions for the patient, either directly by withholding information about options or indirectly by voicing recommendations in a way that leaves little room for questioning or disagreeing.

The traditional argument in favor of parentalism takes two forms, both presupposing the incompetence of sick people. One is based on the clearly false assumption that all sick people, because of pain, fear, and anxiety, are incompetent to make decisions for themselves and, furthermore, do not want to do so. While this may be true for some people, and more true in the past than at present, it applies only infrequently to a woman at the age of menopause who may not see herself as "sick" at all.

The second argument for parentalism is a stronger one, beginning with Plato's insight that the practice of any art, including the art of medicine, depends on having specialized knowledge. By contrast, the nonprofessional, that is, the patient, does not have such knowledge and thus cannot understand or appreciate the technicalities of medicine. Good decision making, the argument continues, requires understanding the specialized knowledge of the profession, and thus, the argument concludes, only the medical professional can make good medical decisions.

This argument is persuasive where there is definitive specialized knowledge. But does it apply when even the qualified professionals are uncertain about what works best and disagree about what to do?

The Nature of Clinical Judgment

One of the major decisions faced by menopausal women concerns the use of hormone replacement therapy (HRT). However, many questions about HRT need answering. What are its long-term effects? What is its relationship to heart disease, stroke, cancer, and osteoporosis? Is it advisable for all women or only some? Should it be taken for just a short time at onset of menopause or be prescribed for life? Is it worth risking the possibility of uterine cancer in order to reduce the risk of bone fractures?

Using HRT as an example, we can see that there are two features of medical judgments relating to menopause that pose a challenge to the position of the parentalistic physician and require the woman, both practically and morally, to assume the role as primary decision maker.

First, some of the most important decisions about the care of menopausal women must be made under conditions of medical uncertainty and professional disagreement. Second, these decisions involve weighing of risks and benefits, which turn on personal values.

Uncertainty

Even among physicians who subscribe to the same medical model of menopause, there is profound disagreement about prescribing HRT.[2] In part, this rests on the fact that, although the benefits in reducing vasomotor symptoms (hot flashes) can be observed in the short term, other, perhaps more important, benefits and very serious risks can be observed only ten or more years after HRT is initiated. Insofar as widespread use of HRT is fairly recent,[3] its long-term results are not really known.

In a recent evaluation of HRT in the journal *Ob/Gyn,* the author explains that recent studies show that cholesterol concentrations are associated with cardiovascular disease, and there are twenty-three studies that show that postmenopausal estrogen therapy changes cholesterol concentrations favorably. However, estrogen therapy also increases the risk of endometrial cancer, and because the risk of cancer is seen as so unacceptable, both physicians and patients prefer the addition of progesterone. Progesterone, however, has an opposite and unfavorable effect on cholesterol concentration, and "the extent to which progestin therapy thus enhances cardiovascular disease risk in postmenopausal women is currently unknown" (Knopp; see also the papers by MacPherson and Voda, this volume).

There are further problems arising from the lack of definitive research. When there is uncertainty in the factors leading to a clinical judgment, and when the judgment rests on the assessment of probabilities, the physician is subject to systematic errors in decision making (Dawson and Arkes).

Other evidence of the "unscientific" nature of HRT clinical judgments has been documented in an interesting study which compared the decisions about prescribing HRT made by practicing physicians in their usual way with decisions that would be made if they used a theoretical decision-making model (Elstein et al.). Decision theory is an explicit logical approach to decision making under uncertainty, developed to take into account in a structured way all the factors physicians say they consider when making clinical judgments.

A model was constructed for each clinician, using the weights he or she assigned to the various risks and benefits. The clinicians were then presented with twelve cases describing women with different variables of being at risk for, say, fractures. The majority of the physicians, on the basis of clinical judgment arrived at in their usual way, opted against HRT. The decision analytic model, however, indicated that either they should recommend treatment or, at least, consider it a toss-up between treatment and nontreatment.

The authors of this study explain the discrepancy by supposing that the physicians based their judgments on the tendency to try to minimize the most serious risk, namely, the risk of endometrial cancer, regardless of its probability, whereas the formal model took account of the fact that early detection (and presumably successful treatment) of cancer is possible by regular followup.

The implication of this is that, in general, the more errors in judgment to which one is susceptible, the less claim one has to the status of expert. Thus, physicians who must make clinical judgments about HRT under the conditions of uncertainty and disagreement which currently prevail, have only partial claim to the status of knowledge and expertise that might justify their role as primary decision makers. It is the uncertainty of clinical judgments that undermines the authority of the physician, not incompetence or ill will, and the uncertainty in HRT decisions cannot be escaped at present.

Values

Suppose you have an itch and a rash that do not go away. You visit a physician who examines the rash, prescribes an ointment with an unpronounceable name, and tells you how often and how long to apply it. You follow the directions and your rash goes away.

From this kind of example, it is easy to suppose that clinical judgment is totally a matter of knowledge and expertise. But look again. Clinical judgment involves choosing means to achieve desired ends, and ends, themselves, are a matter of choice.

Some ends or goals are so obvious and universal they need not be stated. In other cases, however, goals may conflict and a choice must be made. For example, one may want both long life and good quality of life, but both may not be possible. In still other cases, there may be different means to achieve essentially the same goals, for example, different drugs with different side effects.

Noticing that medical decisions involve choices of goals and sometimes choices between treatments helps us to recognize that medical decisions involve values as well as expertise. If clinical judgment were a matter only of medical expertise, then it would make sense that all decisions should be made by the experts alone. But, since they are not, the case for the physician as primary decision maker is seriously weakened. Physicians are not necessarily experts about values, and my physician certainly is not an expert at knowing or choosing my goals.

If a competent person wants to waive her or his right to decision making, it would make sense to do so only when the substitute decision maker is someone who shares the same values and goals, for example, a fellow member of a religious community with clearly articulated beliefs about medical care. However, doctors and patients most often do not share values. Typically in the United States, there are wide differences in economic and social class, education—and in the case of obstetrics and gynecology, gender—between doctors and patients (Starr chap. 3).

More specifically, there are significant differences between what physicians of menopause-age women think is important, what they think their patients think is important, and what women actually think is important. Some of the differences have been detailed in two recent studies.

In 1987 Holmes et al. interviewed physicians and healthy women and asked them to rank their preferences of various possible long-term outcomes of HRT. Physicians were asked to rank their own preferences and also their estimate of what their women patients would prefer. In general, physicians rated illness episodes followed by recovery as closer to perfect health than the women did. Further, physicians were quite wrong about how women would rank the choice between relief of vasomotor symptoms and fracture prevention. The physicians thought the women would rank relief of symptoms higher, whereas the women actually ranked fracture prevention as more important to them.

The most striking difference was in ranking what could be considered the most extreme outcome, premature postoperative death at age 65. Almost half the women ranked premature death as better than serious prolonged disability from fractures, while only ten percent of the physicians did so. Although the authors do not comment, this result is consistent with the widespread general impression that physicians tend to support life-extending measures whenever possible and tend to attach less value to quality vs. quantity of life than do many patients.

An earlier study compared a group of physicians, practicing nurses, and women of menopausal or postmenopausal age, asking them to rank fifteen symptoms for frequency, severity, and causality and to rate their preferences for treatment through counseling, HRT, mood-altering medication, or no treatment (Cowan et al.). The results of this study, too, indicated significant differences between the rankings of medical professionals and their potential women patients. The physicians and nurses judged the various symptoms to be generally more frequent and more severe than the women did, each woman reporting on her own experience. Even more interestingly, the physicians and nurses used a psychogenic model, attributing symptoms to psychological causes, whereas the women attributed symptoms to somatic, that is, bodily causes. Connected with this, physicians rated HRT more favorably than did either the women or nurses, and were more in favor of counseling than the women or nurses. Both physicians and nurses preferred counseling to hormone treatment, but the women rated counseling and HRT equally. The authors interpret these findings as one more piece of evidence to support the general claim that health-care providers tend to downplay somatic causes in favor of psychogenic causes of female "complaints" (Cowan et al. 11). The authors also conclude from the study that the physicians and nurses did not demonstrate familiarity with the literature showing that women do not dread menopause.

The significant differences between physicians' and women patients' perceptions and preferences concerning menopause are explained by the value component of clinical judgment. Thus, insofar as physicians assume a parentalistic, primary decision-making role, they are imposing their own values on patients who may have quite different values. However well-intentioned this might be, it is profoundly wrong, from a moral point of view.

Rational Choice

Is a woman's choice which reflects a preference for premature death over prolonged disability irrational? What does it mean for a choice to be rational? Can a physician's choice for a woman patient be more rational than her own choice would be? If so, could this then justify parentalism?

The traditional view has been that reason is the same in all human beings, thus what is rational for one person is rational for all. The theory of proxy consent in medicine rests on this assumption. If a mature person becomes incompetent, a guardian may make decisions for her, but should do so using the standard of "substituted judgment," that is, choosing as one thinks that person would choose. However, if one is proxy for an infant or a person who has been profoundly retarded since birth, that is, one who has never been able to form her own values and preferences, then one should choose according to "the reasonable person" standard, that is, what any reasonable person would choose in that same circumstance (President's Commission 136).

Who is this so-called reasonable person? Presumably, a person whose rational capacities are fully developed, but whose choices are independent of any subjective or personal elements, such as age, race, gender, or class. In this way, the morally desirable characteristics of objectivity and universality can be achieved in the decision.

On the "objective" view of the reasonable person, that person is neither child nor retired person. He (typically male) is in midlife, which is considered prime of life, and his values are the values of a person at that stage. Thus, when anyone chooses for another according to a reasonable person standard, one chooses according to prime-of-life values.

However, not all people are at the midlife stage, and it should not be considered irrational for older adults to choose according to a different set of values. Without attempting a sophisticated definition of "rational" here, we may say that the decisions of a competent, informed, uncoerced adult who chooses in accordance with her own perceived needs and preferences should be honored as rational.

We could, then, construct a quite different model of rational choice. On this model, we would use the concept of rationality in such a way that we could say it is rational for people with different characteristics to make different choices for themselves.[4] Specifically, we could say it is rational for people at different ages to choose differently. This model of rational choice allows us to recognize differences due to developmental growth, growth which psychologists now assure us does not end at puberty (Sheehy; Levinson). Adults as well as children pass through life stages, and their needs, preferences, and values change over time.

This concept of rational choice is not entirely subjective. It does not imply that one must honor any choice of any person as rational. It preserves a sense of "irrational" which would apply, say, to the person who is ignorant or misled about the consequences of her choice, who is compelled by fear or pain into a choice that does not fit her own stated goals. But it does include a sense of subjectivity such that what is rational for one person to choose is not necessarily rational for another, dependent on circumstances and personal values.

To take this analysis a step farther: Rational choices vary not only with age but with gender, ethnic or religious background, and economic class, among other things. Thus, the moral dangers and moral wrongness of imposing one's own values on others by making decisions for them multiply. When persons are incompetent or otherwise unable to make decisions for themselves, proxy consent cannot be avoided. But when persons are competent, the importance of empowering individuals to make their own choices according to their own values cannot be emphasized too much.

Conclusion

I have offered an analysis of the particular features of clinical judgments about treatment of menopause-age women which challenge the traditional role of the physician as primary decision maker. Because of the uncertainty about the effectiveness and safety of HRT, because of the way in which choices between treatments involve not only medical expertise but personal values, and because of the gap that exists between what physicians think their women patients want and what women of menopause age themselves say they want, it is imperative that women take an active and determinative role in decision making for themselves.

The implications should be clear, namely, that a change in the typical doctor/patient relationship is needed, moving from a priestly model (Veatch), where the physician speaks from a position of total authority, to a more collegial model, where knowledge and decision making is shared as much as possible.

Insofar as the doctor/patient relationship is a professional one, the two parties will never be completely equal. The woman who consults a physician needs the professional's medical knowledge, experience, and advice. But the context in which that advice is sought and given needs to be changed.

Change in a relationship requires change on both sides. Physicians need to abandon the psychogenic model which is denigrating when applied to menopause-age women as a class. In doing so, they will be abandoning many of the myths they have inherited from past generations of the medical profession. To substitute for the old myths, they need to listen to women's voices about their own experience and explore with each individual patient her own values and preferences.

Similar changes need to be undertaken by those in the patient role. Women must be willing to assert their right to participate in decision making, do the hard work of recognizing and voicing their own values and goals, and, perhaps most difficult of all, be willing to accept responsibility for making their own choices. Making choices can be exhilarating, but it can also be frightening, especially in an unfamiliar area where the results of a bad choice can be serious long-term consequences for one's health and well-being. However, before we can expect others to have a new image of us, we must develop a new image of ourselves. Women must learn to feel and think like decision makers in order to become decision makers.

NOTES

1. Note, though, that widely disparate figures are given of how many women seek medical treatment, with some estimates as low as 10%–30% (Cowan, Warren, and Young).

2. See the papers by Susan Johnson and Kristi Ferguson, and Kathleen MacPherson, this volume.

3. R. Wilson's book, *Feminine Forever*, promoting the use of estrogen replacement (ERT), was published in 1966, and articles suggesting the connection between ERT and endometrial cancer began appearing in the medical journals about 1975. I use "HRT" generically, to refer to estrogen-only and combination drugs. For a fuller discussion of the distinction between ERT and HRT, see the paper by Ann Voda, this volume.

4. My thinking on this topic owes much to Michael Slote, *Goods and Virtues* (New York: Oxford, 1983), chaps. 1 and 2. See also Rosalind Ekman Ladd and Edwin N. Forman, Adolescent decision-making: giving weight to age-specific values, forthcoming in *Theoretical Medicine*.

REFERENCES

Brenner, Paul F. 1988. The menopausal syndrome, *Ob/Gyn* 72:6S.

Cowan, Gloria, L. W. Warren, and J. L Young. 1985 Medical perceptions of menopausal symptoms. *Psychology of Women Quarterly* 9:3–14.

Dawson, Neal, and Hal R. Arkes. 1987. Systematic errors in medical decision making: Judgment limitations. *Journal of General Internal Medicine* 2:183–87.

Ehrenreich, Barbara, and Deirdre English. 1973. *Complaints and Disorders: The Sexual Politics of Sickness.* Old Westbury, N.Y.: Feminist Press.

Elstein, Arthur S., et al. 1986. Comparison of physicians' decisions regarding estrogen replacement therapy for menopausal women and decisions derived from a decision analytic model. *American Journal of Medicine* 80:246–58.

Holmes, Margaret, et al. 1987. Women's and physicians' utilities for health outcomes in ERT. *Journal of General Internal Medicine* 2:178–82.

Knopp, Robert H. 1988. The effects of postmenopausal estrogen therapy on the incidence of arteriosclerotic vascular disease. *OB/Gyn* 72:23S–29S.

Levinson, D. L. 1978. *The Seasons of a Man's Life.* New York: Knopf.

McCrea, Frances. 1983. The politics of menopause: The "discovery" of a deficiency disease. *Social Problems* 31:11–123.

Notman, Malkah T., and Carol C. Nadelson. 1978. The woman patient. In Notman and Nadelson, eds., *The Woman Patient: Medical and Psychological Interfaces* I. 1–7. New York: Plenum.

President's Commission for the Study of Ethical Problems in Medicine and Biomedical and Behavioral Research. 1983. *Deciding to Forego Life-Sustaining Treatment.* Washington, D.C.: U.S. Printing Office.

Sheehy, Gail. 1976. *Passages: Predictable Crises of Adult Life.* New York: Dutton.

Starr, Paul. 1982 *The Social Transformation of American Medicine.* New York: Basic Books.

Veatch, Robert. 1983. Models of ethical medicine in a revolutionary age. In Gorovitz et al., eds., *Moral Problems in Medicine,* 2nd ed., Englewood Cliffs, N.J.: Prentice Hall.

AFTERWORD: CREATING A VISUAL IMAGE OF MENOPAUSE: THE *HOT FLASH FAN*

ANN STEWART ANDERSON

Usually, when artists create works, they draw from a vast reservoir of visual precedents. A figure painter knows Rembrandt and Cassatt, a tomb sculptor is aware of Ramses and Michelangelo.

When we conceived of making a work of art about menopause, it seemed reasonable to start by looking at what other artists had done with this subject. What we found, to our initial dismay and eventual joy, was that although we suspect that women have indeed dealt with this subject in their private journals and needlework, there was no public tradition of menopausal images. Other aspects of female biological events have been the subject of numerous artistic expressions. There are compelling images of woman as a symbol of fertility from prehistoric, wide-hipped, pendulous-breasted figures in clay to the voluptuous Venuses painted by Titian. Representations of rites of passage into puberty abound, with accompanying traditional garments, dwellings, and rituals. Birth has been depicted by many primitive tribes and, most recently, in Judy Chicago's *Birth Project*. But our research revealed that menopause simply does not have a recognized visual tradition.

Starting our research in the library, we found surprisingly few books on menopause. Some medical texts described physiological phenomena, some authors tackled the worries about emotional trauma, while a few dealt with a feminist concept of a freer woman in her new body. There was little anthropological or historical material.

So we did what we should have done from the beginning. We went to women themselves. Devising a questionnaire which dealt with both the reality of and the myths about menopause, we gathered comments as diverse as "the only thing I care less about than adolescence is menopause" to "this was a time in which I found great strength." A woman told of her grandmother who had hit her head against the wall in rage against her hot flashes. Another said that "I really liked my hot flashes! It was winter and wonderfully warming."

We obviously had a subject that is charged with myth and emotion, filled with contradictions, and important to many women.

After we collated the material from the questionnaires and the published material, we began to work on a visual image.

Creating an initial image is an onerous task and a rare challenge. It has to be meaningful; it has to be correct; it has to be an honest and valid first step.

Our research told us that there are many manifestations of menopause, but the one which is virtually universal is the hot flash. And so it was that a fan seemed the most appropriate basis for our design.

Recognizing the essential complexity of our subject, we decided to color the fan like a spectrum: twelve blades hued from warm yellow to cool green, with inserts, in the opposite direction, green to yellow, reading left to right. Based on the information we had gathered, we assigned each section of the fan to an aspect of menopause, drawing on both reality and myth. At the top, each insert is lettered with the words "menopause is."

Reading from the lower left, the first yellow panel represents the lack of interest in sex. A loss of sexual attractiveness accompanying menopause is a feeling often attributed to women.

The second, yellow-orange panel describes the ugly, witch-like images which are often imposed on menopausal women by men and younger women, resulting in female anxieties. They are fears of becoming a middle-aged, overweight shrew, of having a permanent scar, of becoming a dried-up old prune. Women express anxieties about perceived biological uselessness, at actually becoming an empty womb.

Panels three and four, flesh and orange in color, deal directly with the whole issue of aging. The woman depicted is drying up, slowing down, going over the hill.

The next two panels, melon and red, deal with the realities and popular myths about menopause in their specific physical manifestations. Included here are wrinkles, dowager's hump, facial fuzz, aching joints, itching skin, frequent urination, fragile bones. The reality is that certain changes do commonly occur; the myth is that these changes are inevitably terrifying.

Panel seven, magenta, represents the end of childbearing years and the accompanying end of the fear of pregnancy and of the necessity for birth control. It also depicts the end of the mess and bother of menstruation.

The next, lavender and blue, panels depict the spiritual transformation and sense of freedom of the woman in menopause. She experiences a re-birth, a great release, a secret joy.

The tenth and eleventh panels, colored turquoise and aqua, deal with the realities and myths of mental distress in menopause. Although a woman may experience some peculiar feelings, it is the outside world that points to her, accusing her of being strange. She is characterized from the outside as hysterical, morbidly irrational, weepy, unable to think straight or concentrate, nervous and irritable, and dominated by mood swings.

The last panel celebrates women who claim to experience PMZ—post-menopausal zest. They experience an increased sex drive, which is the ultimate result of the freedom of menopause.

A large semicircle, with the words "Hot Flashes" forms the center of the fan.

Many artists worked on this project. People stitched, beaded, embroi-dered, made coffee, organized parking, brought lunch, did research, of-fered ideas. Although the major construction was done in Louisville, women from Massachusetts, Iowa, California, Texas, Pennsylvania, Colo-rado, and New Mexico worked on it. Many talked of their own hot flashes while we worked. Often, as we quilted together, we did what women have always done—we shared our ideas on aging and strengthened ourselves from our conversations and our creating.

For some of us, menopause occurred during the actual fabrication of the *Hot Flash Fan*. Making it became an eminently significant personal rite of passage. This piece, created in collaboration, made by hand, expressing the diversity of traditional myths, historical attitudes, and physical facts, is an important image, significant in woman's history, marking and celebrat-ing, at last, the menopause.

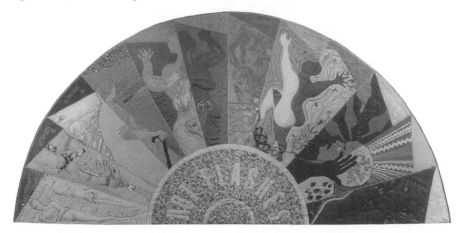

SELECTED INTERDISCIPLINARY BIBLIOGRAPHY ON MENOPAUSE

JILL RIPS

Culturally and Cross-Culturally

Anderst, Moira J. 1975. "Nuns in Menopause: Their Attitudes and Symptoms." Master of Nursing Thesis, University of Washington, Seattle.

"Anthropological Approaches to Menopause: Questioning Received Knowledge." 1986. *Special Issue: Culture, Medicine and Psychiatry* 10(1), Margaret Lock, Guest Editor.

Barnett, Elyse A. 1986. "Perceptions of Menopause: Importance of Role Satisfaction in a Peruvian Town." Doctoral Dissertation, Department of Anthropology, Stanford University, Palo Alto, Calif.

Bart, Pauline. 1969. "Why Women's Status Changes in Middle Age." *Sociological Symposium* 3:1–18.

Bart, Pauline, and Grossman, M. 1976. "Menopause." *Women and Health* 1:3–11.

Beyene, Yewoubdar. 1984. "An Ethnography of Menopause: Menopausal Experience of Mayan Women in a Yucatan Village." Doctoral Dissertation, Department of Anthropology, Case Western Reserve University, Cleveland.

———. 1986. "Cultural Significance and Physiological Manifestations of Menopause: A Biocultural Analysis." *Culture, Medicine and Psychiatry* 10(1): 47–71.

———. 1989. *From Menarche to Menopause: Reproductive Lives of Peasant Women in Two Cultures.* Albany: State University of New York Press.

Brooks-Gunn, Jeanne. 1982. "A Sociocultural Approach." In *Changing Perspectives on Menopause,* ed. Ann M. Voda, Myra Dinnerstein, and Sheryl R. O'Donnell, 203–208. Austin: University of Texas Press.

Brown, Judith K., and Kerns, Virginia, eds. 1985. *In Her Prime: A New View of Middle-Aged Women.* South Hadley, Mass.: Bergen and Garvey.

Datan, Nancy; Antonovsky, Aaron; and Moaz, Benjamin. 1981. *A Time to Reap: The Middle Age of Women in Five Israeli Subcultures.* Baltimore: Johns Hopkins University Press.

Davis, Dona Lee. 1982. "Women's Status and Experience of the Menopause in a Newfoundland Fishing Village." *Maturitas* 4:207–16.

———. 1983. *Nerves and Blood: An Ethnographic Focus on Menopause.* St. John's: Memorial University of Newfoundland.

Dougherty, Molly. 1978. "An Anthropological Perspective on Aging and Women in the Middle Years." In *The Anthropology of Health,* ed. Eleanor E. Bauwens, 167–76. St. Louis: C. V. Mosby.

Dowty, N.; Maoz, B.; Antonovsky, A.; and Wijsenbeek, H. 1970. "Climacterium in Three Cultural Contexts." *Tropical and Geographical Medicine* 22:77–86.

du Toit, Brian. 1990. *Aging and Menopause among Indian South African Women.* New York: State University of New York Press.

Flint, Marcha. 1974. "Menarche and Menopause of Rajput Women." Doctoral Dissertation, Department of Anthropology, City University of New York.

———. 1975. "The Menopause: Reward or Punishment?" *Psychosomatics* 16:161–63.

———. 1982. "Anthropological Perspectives on the Menopause and Middle Age." *Maturitas* 4:173–80.

Flint, Marcha, and Garcia, M. 1979. "Culture and the Climacteric." *Journal of Biosocial Science, Supplement* 6:197–215.

George, Theresa. 1985. "There Is a Time for Everything: A Study of the Menopausal/Climacteric Experience of Sikh Women in Canada." Doctoral Dissertation, Department of Anthropology, University of Utah, Salt Lake City.

Goodman, M. J.; Stewart, C. J.; and Gilbert, F. 1977. "Patterns of Menopause: A Study of Certain Medical and Physiological Variables among Caucasian and Japanese Women Living in Hawaii." *Journal of Gerontology* 32(3):291–98.

Griffen, J. 1977. "A Cross-Cultural Investigation of Behavioral Changes at Menopause." *The Social Science Journal* 14(2):49–55.

———. 1982. "Cultural Models for Coping with Menopause." In *Changing Perspectives on Menopause,* ed. Ann M. Voda, Myra Dinnerstein, and Sheryl R. O'Donnell, 249–62. Austin: University of Texas Press.

Kaufert, Patricia. 1982. "Anthropology and the Menopause: The Development of a Theoretical Framework." *Maturitas* 4:181–93.

———. 1985. "Midlife in the Midwest: Canadian Women in Manitoba." In *In Her Prime: A New View of Middle-Aged Women,* ed. Judith K. Brown and Virginia Kerns, 181–97. South Hadley, Mass.: Bergen and Garvey.

Kaufert, Patricia; Lock, Margaret; McKinlay, Sonja; et al. 1986. "Menopause Research: The Korpilampi Workshop." *Social Science and Medicine* 22 (11):1285–89.

Kay, M.; Voda, A.; Olivas, G.; Rios, I.; and Imle, M. 1982. "Ethnography of the Menopause-Related Hot Flash." *Maturitas* 4:217–27.

Kearnes, Bessie J. R. 1982. "Perceptions of Menopause by Papago Women." In *Changing Perspectives on Menopause,* ed. Ann M. Voda, Myra Dinnerstein, and Sheryl R. O'Donnell, 70–83. Austin: University of Texas Press.

Lancaster, Jane B., and King, Barbara J. 1985. "An Evolutionary Perspective on Menopause." In *In Her Prime: A New View of Middle-Aged Women,* ed. Judith K. Brown and Virginia Kerns, 13–20. South Hadley, Mass.: Bergen and Garvey.

Lock, Margaret. 1988. "New Japanese Mythologies: Faltering Discipline and the Ailing Housewife." *American Ethnologist: Special Issue on Medical Anthropology* 15(1):43–60.

Lock, Margaret; Kaufert, Patricia; and Gilbert, Penny. 1988. "Cultural Construction of the Menopausal Syndrome: The Japanese." *Maturitas* 10:317–32.

Martin, Emily. 1987. "Medical Metaphors of Women's Bodies: Menstruation and Menopause." In *The Woman in the Body: A Cultural Analysis of Reproduction,* 27–53. Boston: Beacon.

Moore, B. 1981. "Climacteric Symptoms in an African Community." *Maturitas* 3:28–29.

210   Selected Interdisciplinary Bibliography

Rosenberger, N. R. 1987. "Productivity, Sexuality and Ideologies of Menopausal Problems in Japan." In *Health, Illness, and Medical Care in Japan: Cultural and Social Dimensions,* ed. Edward Norbeck and Margaret Lock, 155–88. Honolulu: University of Hawaii Press.

Sharma, V. K., and Saxena, M. S. L. 1981. "Climacteric Symptoms: A Study in the Indian Context." *Maturitas* 3:11–20.

Silverman, Sydel F. 1975. "The Life Crisis as a Clue to Social Function: The Case of Italy." In *Toward an Anthropology of Women,* ed. Rayna R. Reiter, 309–21. New York: Monthly Review.

Skultans, Vieda. 1970. "The Symbolic Significance of Menstruation and Menopause." *Man* 5(4):639–51.

———. 1989. "Menstrual Symbolism in South Wales." In *Blood Magic: The Anthropology of Menstruation,* ed. Thomas Buckley and Alma Gottlieb, 137–60. Berkeley: University of California Press.

Wilbush, Joel. 1985. "Surveys of Climacteric Semiology in non-Western Populations: A Critique." *Maturitas* 7:289–96.

Somatic and Psychiatric Epidemiology and Physiology: Symptom Reporting and Health-Care Utilization

Bowles, C. 1986. "Measure of Attitude toward Menopause Using the Semantic Differential Model." *Nursing Research* 35(2):81–85.

Dennerstein, Lorraine, and Burrows, Graham D. 1978. "A Review of Studies of the Psychological Symptoms Found at the Menopause." *Maturitas* 1:55–64.

Engle, N. S. 1987. "Menopausal Stage, Current Life Change, Attitude toward Women's Roles, and Perceived Health Status." *Nursing Research* 36 (6):353–57.

Feldman, B.; Voda, A.; and Gronseth, E. 1985. "The Prevalence of Hot Flash and Associated Variables among Perimenopausal Women." *Research in Nursing and Health* 8:261–68.

Frey, Karen A. 1982. "Middle-Aged Women's Experience and Perceptions of Menopause." *Women and Health* 6(1/2):25–35.

Greene, John Gerald. 1984. *The Social and Psychological Origins of the Climacteric Syndrome.* Brookfield, Vt.: Gower.

Kaufert, Patricia. 1980. "The Menopausal Woman and Her Use of Health Services." *Maturitas* 2:191–206.

———. 1988. "Menopause as Process or Event: The Creation of Definitions in Biomedicine." In *Biomedicine Examined,* ed. Margaret Lock and Deborah R. Gordon, 331–49. Norwell, Mass.: Kluwer.

Kaufert, Patricia, and Gilbert, Penny. 1986a. "The Context of Menopause: Psychotropic Drug Use and Menopausal Status." *Social Science and Medicine* 23(8):747–55.

———. 1986b. "Women, Menopause and Medicalization." *Culture, Medicine and Psychiatry* 10:7–21.

Kaufert, Patricia, and Syrotuik, J. 1981. "Symptom Reporting at the Menopause." *Social Science and Medicine* 15E:173–84.

LaRocco, S., and Polit, D. 1980. "Women's Knowledge about the Menopause." *Nursing Research* 29(1):10–13.

Lennon, Mary Clare. 1980. "Psychological Reactions to Menopause: A Sociological Study." Doctoral Dissertation, Department of Sociology, Columbia University, New York.

———. 1982. "The Psychological Consequences of Menopause: The Importance of Timing of a Life Stage Event." *Journal of Health and Social Behavior* 23:353–66.

Maoz, Benjamin; Antonovsky, Aaron; Apter, Alan; et al. 1978. "The Effect of Outside Work on the Menopausal Woman." *Maturitas* 1:42–53.

Maoz, B.; Dowty, N.; Antonovsky, A.; and Wysjenbeek, H. 1970. "Female Attitudes to Menopause." *Social Psychiatry* 1:35–40.

Martin, Emily. 1987. "Menopause, Power and Heat." In *The Woman in the Body: A Cultural Analysis of Reproduction,* 166–78. Boston: Beacon.

McKinlay, Sonja. 1988. "The Impact of Menopause and Social Factors on Health." In *Menopause: Evaluation, Treatment and Health Concerns,* ed. C. Hammond, F. Haseltin, and I. Schiff. New York: Alan Liss.

McKinlay, Sonja, and McKinlay, John. 1973. "Selected Studies of the Menopause: An Annotated Bibliography." *Journal of Biosocial Science* 5:533–55.

———. 1985. "Health Status and Health Care Utilization by Menopausal Women." In *Aging, Reproduction and the Climacteric,* 213–62. New York: Plenum.

McKinlay, John; McKinlay, Sonja; and Brambilla, Donald J. 1987a. "Health Status and Utilization Behavior Associated with Menopause." *American Journal of Epidemiology* 125(1):110–21.

———. 1987b. "The Relative Contributions of Endocrine Changes and Social Circumstances to Depression in Mid-Aged Women." *Journal of Health and Social Behavior* 28:345–63.

Millette, B. M. 1981. "Menopause: A Survey of Attitudes and Knowledge." *Issues in Health Care of Women* 3:263–76.

Neugarten, Bernice, et al. 1963. "Women's Attitudes toward the Menopause." *Vita Humana* 6:140–51.

Polit, D. F., and LaRocco, S. A. 1980. "Social and Psychological Correlates of Menopause Symptoms." *Psychosomatic Medicine* 42(3):335–45.

Uphold, C. R., and Susman, E. J. 1981. "Self-reported Climacteric Symptoms." *Nursing Research* 30(2):84–88.

Woods, N. F. 1982. "Menopausal Distress: A Model for Epidemiologic Investigation." In *Changing Perspectives on Menopause,* ed. Ann M. Voda, Myra Dinnerstein, and Sheryl R. O'Donnell, 220–38. Austin: University of Texas Press.

Historically, Politically, Economically

Delaney, J.; Lupton, M. J.; and Toth, E. 1976. "From Leeches to Estrogen: The Menopause and Medical Options," "Psychology and the Menopausal Menace," and "November of the Body: The Menopause and Literature." In *The Curse: A Cultural History of Menstruation,* 177–200. New York: Dutton.

Grossman, M., and Bart, P. 1979. "Taking Men out of Menopause." In *Women Looking at Biology Looking at Women,* ed. Ruth Hubbard, M. S. Henifin, and B. Fried, 163–84. Boston: Hall.

Kaufert, Patricia, and McKinlay, Sonja. 1985. "Estrogen Replacement Therapy: The Production of Medical Knowledge and the Emergence of Policy." In *Women Health and Healing: Toward a New Perspective,* ed. Ellen Lewin and Virginia Olesen, 113–38. London: Tavistock.

Laws, Sophie. 1990. *Issues of Blood: The Politics of Menstruation.* Houndmills, England: Macmillan.

Lennon, Mary Clare. 1980. "The Nineteenth Century View of Menopause."

"Psychological Reactions to Menopause: A Sociological Study." Doctoral Dissertation, Department of Sociology, Columbia University, New York.
MacPherson, Kathleen I. 1986. "Feminist Praxis in the Making: The Menopause Collective." Doctoral Dissertation, Department of Sociology, Brandeis University, Boston.
McCrea, F. B. 1983. "The Politics of Menopause: The 'Discovery' of a Deficiency Disease." *Social Problems* 31(1):111–23.
Mitteness, Linda S. 1983. "Historical Changes in Public Information about the Menopause." *Urban Anthropology* 12(2):161–79.
Smith-Rosenberg, Carroll. 1973. "Puberty to Menopause: The Cycle of Femininity in Nineteenth-Century America." *Feminist Studies* 1(3/4):58–73.
Wilbush, Joel. 1981. "What's in a Name?: Some Linguistic Aspects of the Climacteric." *Maturitas* 3:1–9.
———. 1982. "Climacteric Expression and Social Context." *Maturitas* 4:195–205.
———. 1988. "Menorrhagia and Menopause: A Historical Review." *Maturitas* 10:5–26.
———. 1989. "Menopause and Menorrhagia: A Historical Exploration." *Maturitas* 10:83–108.

Social Construction of Menopausal Models

Dickson, G. 1990. "A Feminist Poststructuralist Analysis of the Knowledge of Menopause." *Advances in Nursing Science* 12(3):15–31.
Kaufert, Patricia. 1982. "Myth and the Menopause." *Sociology of Health and Illness* 4(2):141–66.
Kaufert, Patricia, and McKinlay, Sonja. 1985. "Estrogen-replacement Therapy: The Production of Medical Knowledge and the Emergence of Policy." In *Women, Health and Healing: Toward a New Perspective,* ed. Ellen Lewin and Virginia Olesen, 113–38. London: Tavistock.
Lock, Margaret. 1982. "Models and Practice in Medicine: Menopause as Syndrome or Life Transition?" *Culture, Medicine and Psychiatry* 6(3):261–80.
MacPherson, Kathleen I. 1981. "Menopause as Disease: The Social Construction of a Metaphor." *Advances in Nursing Science* 3(2):95–113.
———. 1985. "Osteoporosis and Menopause: A Feminist Analysis of the Social Construction of a Syndrome." *Advances in Nursing Science* 7(4):11–22.
Posner, Judith. 1979. "It's All in Your Head: Feminist and Medical Models of Menopause (Strange Bedfellows)." *Sex Roles* 5(2):179–90.
Townsend, John M., and Carbone, Cynthia L. 1980. "Menopausal Syndrome: Illness or Social Role—A Transcultural Analysis." *Culture, Medicine and Psychiatry* 4:229–48.

Self-Help Guides for Menopause Utilizing a Nonmedicalized Perspective

Costolow, J.; Lopez, M. C.; and Taub, M. 1989. *Menopause: A Self-care Manual.* Sante Fe: Santa Fe Health Education Project.
Doress, P. D., and Siegal, D. L. 1987. *Ourselves, Growing Older.* New York: Simon and Schuster.
Gerson, Miryam, and Byrne-Hunter, Rosemary. 1988. *A Book about Menopause.* Montreal: Montreal Health.
National Women's Health Network. 1989. *Taking Hormones and Women's*

Health: Choices, Risks and Benefits. Washington, D.C.: National Women's
Health Network.

Reitz, Rosetta. 1977. *Menopause: A Positive Approach.* New York: Penguin.

Seaman, Barbara, and Seaman, Gideon. 1977. "ERT: Promise Her Anything but
Give Her . . . Cancer" and "Menopause: Wholesome Remedies." In
Women and the Crisis in Sex Hormones, 337–511. New York: Bantam.

Sheehy, Gail. 1991. "The Silent Passage: Menopause." *Vanity Fair,* October: 222–
27, 252, 254, 256, 258, 260–63.

Voda, Ann M. 1984. *Menopause, Me and You: A Personal Handbook for Women.*
Salt Lake City: University of Utah College of Nursing.

Weideger, Paula. 1975. *Menstruation and Menopause: The Physiology and Psychology, the Myth and the Reality.* New York: Dell.

Wilson, Jeanie. 1990. "Estrogen after Menopause: Are the Rewards Worth the
Risk?" *Town and Country,* Oct.: 223–26, 297, 298.

Personal Accounts and Experiences of Menopause

Downing, C. 1989. *Journey through Menopause: A Personal Rite of Passage.* New
York: Crossroad.

Logothetis, Mary Lou. 1991. "Our Legacy: Medical Views of the Menopausal
Woman." In *Women of the Fourteenth Moon: Writings on Menopause,* ed.
D. Taylor and A. Sumrall, 40–46. Watsonville, Calif.: Crossing.

Mankowitz, A. 1984. *Change of Life: A Psychological Study of Dreams and the
Menopause.* Toronto: Inner City.

Taylor, D. 1988. "Menopause: Last Blood." In *Red Flower: Rethinking Menstruation,* 92–106. Watsonville, Calif.: Crossing.

Positive Images of Midlife Women in Literature

Arnold, June. 1975. *Sister Gin.* New York: Feminist Press at the City University of
New York.

Gullette, Margaret Morganroth. 1988. *Safe at Last in the Middle Years—The Invention of the Midlife Progress Novel: Saul Bellow, Margaret Drabble, Anne
Tyler, and John Updike.* Berkeley: University of California.

Laurence, Margaret. 1974. *The Diviners.* New York: Knopf.

Lessing, Doris. 1973. *The Summer before the Dark.* New York: Knopf.

Positive Images of Midlife Women in Film

Aviad, Michal. 1987. *Acting Our Age.* Los Angeles: Direct Cinema.

Billops, Camille. 1987. *Older Women and Love.* New York: Women Make Movies.

Ranier, Yvonne. 1990. *Privilege.* New York: Zeitgeist Films.

Wynn, Sabina. 1989. *Invisible Women.* New York: Women Make Movies.

CONTRIBUTORS

ANN STEWART ANDERSON is a visual artist. Her work is exhibited in New York, Chicago, Atlanta, and Kentucky and has been supported by grants from the Kentucky Foundation for Women and New Forms Regional Institute.

JOY WEBSTER BARBRE is a graduate student in American Studies and the Center for Advanced Feminist Studies at the University of Minnesota. She is one of the editors of *Interpreting Women's Lives: Feminist Theory and Personal Narratives* and is currently completing a dissertation on the cultural history of menopause in America.

CAROLYN S. BRATT is W. L. Matthews Professor of Law at the University of Kentucky. In addition to her specialization in property law, her research, writing, and teaching have focused on legal issues relating to gender.

JOAN C. CALLAHAN is Associate Professor of Philosophy at the University of Kentucky. She is author of a number of articles in ethics and social philosophy, and she is editor of *Ethical Issues in Professional Life.* Her recent work has focused on reproduction and includes *Preventing Birth: Contemporary Methods and Related Moral Controversies,* coauthored with reproductive physiologist James W. Knight. She is currently working on a collection of new essays, *Reproduction, Ethics, and the Law: Feminist Perspectives.*

GERI L. DICKSON teaches nursing at New York University and is the author of a number of papers and articles on nursing theory, wellness, and menopause.

KRISTI J. FERGUSON is Associate Research Scientist at the University of Iowa College of Medicine. Her research interests pertain to how individuals' perceptions about a given recommendation influence their health-related behavior. She is coinvestigator with Susan R. Johnson on a survey of women's knowledge of menopause, women's attitudes toward menopause, and women's decision making on hormone replacement.

SUSAN R. JOHNSON, M.D., is Director of the Menopause Clinic at the University of Iowa Hospitals and Clinics. She is coinvestigator with Kristi J. Ferguson on a survey of women's knowledge of menopause, women's attitudes toward menopause, and women's decision making on hormone replacement. She is also a coinvestigator in the NIH-sponsored Postmenopausal Estrogen/Progestin Intervention Trial (PEPI).

JEAN KOZLOWSKI is a freelance writer and a member of the Dramatists' Guild.

ROSALIND EKMAN LADD is Professor of Philosophy at Wheaton College and Lecturer in Pediatrics at Brown University Medical School. Her recent works include *Ethical Dilemmas in Pediatrics: A Case Study Approach,* with E. N. Forman, and "Women in Labor: Some Issues About Informed Consent," in *Feminist Perspectives in Medical Ethics,* edited by Helen Bequaert Holmes and Laura M. Purdy.

MARY LOU LOGOTHETIS has been Associate Professor of Parent-Child Nursing and Women's Health in the College of Nursing at Valparaiso University for twelve years. She has over twenty years of experience in a variety of roles related to the health care of women, with special interest in the menstrual cycle and its effects on women's lives. Her recent publications include: "Women's Decisions About Estrogen Replacement Therapy," *Western Journal of Nursing Research,* and "Our Legacy: Medical Views of the Menopausal Woman," in *Women of the 14th Moon: Writings on Menopause,* edited by D. Taylor and A. Sumrall.

KATHLEEN I. MACPHERSON is Professor of Nursing at the University of Southern Maine. She is a women's movement activist and author of feminist articles on menopause and osteoporosis.

JILL RIPS is a doctoral candidate in Sociomedical Sciences at Columbia University. She is an adjunct instructor for Columbia University's School of Public Health in the areas of medical anthropology and women's health. Her research interests are in social constructions of the body, of diseases, and, in particular, of menopause. Currently, as part of an AIDS treatment center in New York, she develops health education curricula and provides technical assistance to peer support groups for inmates and homeless persons who are HIV-positive.

PATRICIA SMITH is Associate Professor and Chair of the Department of Philosophy at the University of Kentucky. She has written in the areas of legal philosophy, social philosophy, and ethics, especially on negligence and responsibility, action theory, and constitutional interpretation. She is editor of *Feminist Jurisprudence* and *The Nature and Process of Law.*

ANN M. VODA is Professor of Nursing at the University of Utah and Director of the Tremin Trust Women's Health Research Foundation, where she is currently directing a longitudinal study, ongoing for 56 years, on menstruation, reproduction, and menopause.

JACQUELYN N. ZITA is Associate Professor of Women's Studies at the University of Minnesota. She has also taught at Webster University, Washington University, Uppsala University, and Michigan State University. She has published numerous essays on theorizing the body in *Hypatia, Signs, Genders, Enclitic,* and *Sinister Wisdom* and is currently completing a collection of writings, *Textualities of Soma.*

INDEX